BULLETPROOF PRIVACY

How to Live Hidden, Happy, and Free!

by

Boston T. Party

Published by

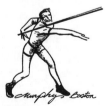

JAVELIN PRESS

c/o P.O. Box 31C, Ignacio, Colorado. (81137-0031)
(Without any 4 USC §§ 105-110 *"Federal area"* or *"State."*)
www.javelinpress.com

DISCLAIMER

Bulletproof Privacy is sold for educational and informational purposes only, and nothing herein is to be considered professional or legal advice. The Author and Publisher disclaim any and all responsibility for liability or loss incurred as a consequence of the use or application, directly and indirectly, of any information presented herein.

First Edition: *January, 1997*
Printed in the united states of America,
without any 4 USC §§ 105-110 *"Federal area"* or *"State."*

10

ISBN 1-888766-02-6

www.javelinpress.com

ACKNOWLEDGMENTS

I thank all my distributors and readers who so enthusiastically have supported my other five books, *Good-Bye April 15th!*, *You & The Police!*, *Hologram of Liberty*, *Boston on Surviving Y2K*, and *Boston's Gun Bible* (an 848pp. behemoth revised in 2002 with over 200 new pages).

DEDICATION

I dedicate *Bulletproof Privacy* to the Liberty-strangling officials of our Federal Government and their hidden masters. Your actions are quickly awakening that sleeping giant—the American spirit—and for that, I thank you.

By all means, continue to *"sow the wind"* that you may *"reap the whirlwind."* I realize that you scoff at any judgment for your actions because American Patriots are rubes. Good. I'm glad that you're haughty—please don't change.

I urge Congress, the President, the courts, and federal agents to *escalate your oppression*, so that America becomes *so* nauseous of tyranny that she finally vomits you out. You have much to accomplish soon, so get on with it. The sooner Americans see you for what you are, the better.

You will soon overstep yourselves. Tyrants always do. You're confident that you've got it all worked out, that you see where Nero and Hitler and Stalin failed. I'm delighted that you believe your "New World Order" plan to be infallible. It's not infallible—for either of two reasons.

❶ Popular resistance will defeat you, or...

❷ Even if you *do* get your NWO, you'll rot from boredom by having such utter control. The "fun" of tyranny isn't in *being* the conqueror, but in the *conquering itself.* (Just ask Alexander the Great.) Lose or "win"—*you've already lost!*

In the long run, you really aren't all that *smart,* are you?

Works by Boston T. Party:

Good-Bye April 15th!

The untaxation classic—crystal clear and sweeping. Copied, plagiarized, and borrowed from, but never equaled. The most effective and least hazardous untaxation guide. Proven over 12 years and thousands of readers!

    392 pp. softcover (1992) $40 + $6 s&h (cash, please)

You & The Police!   (revised for 2005)

The definitive guide to your rights and tactics during police confrontations. When can you *refuse* to answer questions or consent to searches? Don't lose your liberty through ignorance! This 2005 edition covers the *USA PATRIOT Act* and much more.

    168 pp. softcover (2005) $16 + $5 s&h (cash, please)

Bulletproof Privacy
How to Live Hidden, Happy, and Free!

Explains precisely how to lay low and be left alone by the snoops, government agents and bureaucrats. Boston shares many of his own unique methods. The bestselling privacy book in America!

    160 pp. softcover (1997) $16 + $5 s&h (cash, please)

Hologram of Liberty
The Constitution's Shocking Alliance
with Big Government   by Kenneth W. Royce

The Convention of 1787 was the most brilliant and subtle *coup d'état* in history. The nationalist framers *designed* a strong government, guaranteed through purposely ambiguous verbiage. Many readers say this is Boston's best book. A jaw-dropper.

    262 pp. softcover (1997) $20 + $5 s&h (cash, please)

Boston on Surviving Y2K
And Other Lovely Disasters

Even though Y2K was Y2¿*Qué*? this title remains highly useful for all preparedness planning. **Now on sale for 50% off!** (It's the same book as The Military Book Club's *Surviving Doomsday*.)

    352 pp. softcover (1998) only $11 + $5 s&h (in cash)

Boston's Gun Bible (new text for 2005)

A rousing how-to/*why*-to on modern gun ownership. Firearms are *"liberty's teeth"* and it's time we remembered it. Fully revised in 2002 with 10 new chapters. ***200+ new pages* were added!** Much more complete than the 2000 edition. No other general gun book is more thorough or useful! Indispensable!

    848 pp. softcover (2002) $28 + $6 s&h (cash, please)

Molôn Labé!   (Boston's first novel)

If you liked *Unintended Consequences* by John Ross and Ayn Rand's *Atlas Shrugged*, then Boston's novel will be a favorite. It dramatically outlines an innovative recipe for Liberty which could actually work! A thinking book for people of action; an action book for people of thought. A freedom classic!

    454 pp. softcover (2004) $24 + $6 s&h (cash, please)
    limited edition hardcover $44 + $6 (while supplies last)

www.javelinpress.com
www.freestatewyoming.org

TABLE OF CONTENTS

12 Privacy With Pagers

13 Your Private Home

14 Privacy & Your Guns

15 A Quiet Living

INTRODUCTION

The modern socialist State is premised on this presupposition: that all things belong to the State, but a portion of this State-owned capital is temporarily leased to private individuals and organizations. This view of the State has influenced much of modern democratic theory.

The free-market-constitutional view of the State is that it is under legal restraints, that the citizen is the sovereign of the legal order, and that whatever authority which citizens have not formally delegated to the State belongs to them.

The battle over the rights of privacy should be seen in light of these two incompatible views of man and the State. *It is a battle over the definition of what constitutes criminal behavior.*

    -- Dr. Gary North; foreword to Mark Nestmann's *How To Achieve Personal and Financial Privacy In A Public Age*

WHAT I *CAN'T* DISCUSS TOO MUCH

Because of the general nature of *Bulletproof Privacy*, I cannot very deeply discuss certain topics which deserve their own books: ID's, computer security, trusts and complex financial tactics--to mention a few. These matters are also highly dynamic given the changing technology and legal climate. Stay up to date and don't rely on stale information.

MY GOAL FOR YOU

What I *can* do for you is fill in the cracks between existing privacy books. For example, nobody to my knowledge has plainly and *explicitly* described what it takes to change domiciles for privacy's sake. Nobody has outlined *precisely* how *not* use the telephones and the mail. I've used at least some variants of privacy measures since junior high school. There probably aren't very many Americans (outside of wanted criminals) who have lived privacy as much as I have. This is not to brag; it's just something I've grown competent at.

At the possible risk to some of my own privacy, I have decided to share much of this knowledge and experience with you. I can't divulge *all* of my tricks, but there's enough here to be of good value to you.

SOME COMMENTS ON THIS BOOK

Unfortunately, the subject matter of privacy does not lend itself to a perfectly seamless and consecutive presentation. For example, talk of a private domicile must simultaneously include discussion of the phone, mail, etc. Thus, perfect organization of a dozen highly interrelated chapters is impossible. I arranged this book as best I could, and the result is at least tolerable. If I don't seem to cover an issue, it's likely that I've addressed it in another chapter. (If not, then write me.)

> *Quotations are in this form.* *Any original emphasis is underlined.* **Any added emphasis of mine is in boldface.** *Omitted text is always replaced by ellipsis (...). When I supplement a quote, my nonitalicized comments are within ( ) or [ ]--(like this, for example).*

Finally, I know in advance that I've left out dozens of useful tidbits--stuff that will begin to come to me the day after the final typesetting. I've lived the private life for *so* long that its familiarity defies an effortless expression. *Bulletproof Privacy* has so far been the book most written *by* me, rather than researched and collated. In fact, 90% of it came right out of my head without reference to any material whatsoever--a diary of knowledge, if you will. After some 160 pages, I judged the book to be complete enough to publish--especially given the urgency of the times. I'd rather you have 85% of what I can offer *now*, versus 99% in 1998, when it will not be as implementable. There is a shockingly short half-life to this kind of information, so use it *quickly*. As the old French saying goes:

Live happy. Live hidden.

Perhaps we will one day have a society less larded by laziness, envy, greed and vociferous government. This won't be for quite a while. Much will have to occur before that's even remotely possible. Until then, keep your assets hidden and your principles cautiously visible. As they used to say in the Balkans, *"Tell the truth and run."* Run and hide so that you may speak the truth another day--*until backed into a corner...*

WHY PRIVACY?

Far from the madding crowd's ignoble strife.
-- Thomas Gray

Here are the Top Six Reasons why individuals want to preserve their privacy:

- ❻ **High-pressure salesmen and "legal fraud."**
- ❺ **The increasing threat of burglary and violent crime.**
- ❹ **Divorce, family disputes, and lawsuits.**
- ❸ **Gossip and false information.**
- ❷ **Political, religious, and racial persecution.**

And the Number One Reason?

Oppressive government, high taxes, and war.

To stop terrorism and organized crime, the American people must give up some of their personal freedom and privacy.
-- Janet "For-The-Kids" Reno

[The] *"disappearing" of individuals is obviously discomforting to institutions and governments determined to control personal activities in the Land of the Free.* **To them it appears downright seditious, since in reality their power depends directly on the number of people they can control...**
-- *100 Ways to Disappear and Live Free*; Eden Press, p. 3

Janet Reno asking us to give up *"some"* of our personal freedom and privacy is like a child molester asking a young girl to give up *"some"* of her virginity. The federal camel is never satisfied with just his *nose* under the tent--he wants to climb in bed, too.

To those who think there's no need for quality privacy; that I'm being wholly ridiculous, just stay home in your sheep pen and wait for the rude knock on your door when you at last bleat that the shearing is too close for comfort. By then, it'll be too late to do anything but sit still and take it.

Hey, wake up! It's the '90's! Let's have no more sappy fantasies. Only 10 states explicitly recognize the right to privacy in their constitutions. The Federal Government treats you like a rented mule and takes a *third* of your life. Under intentionally contradictory regulations, you're damned if you and damned if you don't, and it's "eeney-meeney-miney-mo" on who gets to seize your property. Will it be IRS, DEA, FBI, U.S. Customs or OSHA? H.R. 666 will kill the 4th Amendment-- now, the feds don't need no stinking search warrant! Thanks to the detailed census form you so helpfully completed about your house and life-style, FEMA will know just how to find you.

LET ME SPELL IT OUT FOR YOU

Gun ownership

This is about to become a real "no-no." Ammo will be taxed out of retail existence. Scoped, bolt-action rifles will become the next bogeyman of the liberals, *"We gotta ban them 'sniper' rifles!"* Got a concealed handgun permit? Well, you'll be real surprised to soon realize that all that wonderful *"shall issue"* CCW legislation was in actuality mere cheese in the mousetrap of eventual confiscation. Sure, they let you carry concealed *now*--they just wanted to learn the *names* of those Americans *serious* enough to do so. (Ancient Chinese proverb: *"Fish see the bait, but not the hook."*) Your CCW permit just got you on a nice little list, along with several million others. (I'd stash the bulk of your gun collection for a rainy decade. The raids are coming.)

Homeschooling

This and spanking your own children will be outlawed by the *U.N. Convention on the Rights of the Child.* Eventually, children will be tattling on their parents. (Recall the daughter who turned in her pot-smoking parents.) Read or watch George Orwell's *1984.* Get to the country while you can, and put a boot through your TV before it mentally, morally plunders your children.

Globe, Inc.

The big corporations are international whores, looking to bed with slave labor wherever it may be found. And who *pays* for the trick? Well, the *slaves* can't afford it, so *we* do--as simpering economic voyeurs. We ghoulishly preside over own destruction. Today, corporations are like station-wagon sized carp--they no longer have any natural enemies (since they now run the government) and they're practically immortal. Watch *Network* and *Rollerball* back to back sometime.

Television--the visual brain cancer

A vulgar, purulent woman has a hit show while networks won't touch the Desert Storm Syndrome.

Our nation now has the approximate literacy rate of Guatemala. **Language missionaries from Nigeria and Pakistan come *here* to teach *English*.** Half of adult Americans believe that criminal suspects are guilty until proven innocent, and only one-third can correctly identify the Bill of Rights. **One-fifth of Americans don't know who won WWII!** For those interested, it was *Japan*. She plunders our pine forests, and modern high-school textbooks no longer mention Pearl Harbor, much less the Bataan Death March.

Ever wonder *why* they call it TV *"programming"*?

Human integrity

You might as well look for Spanish doubloons at the beach. The concept of the *gentleman* is over and gone. True story: gorgeous, utterly faithful Wife travels out of town with her two beautiful children, and she's no sooner down the street than Husband begins plotting his glorious night out at the skankiest topless bar he can manage to find through a sodden bourbon haze.

Men, if you have a loyal woman who loves you, you'd better praise her to the stars and back for what a treasure she is in your life. Without the ladies, we stare into the gray, stupid, canine abyss of ourselves, and those of you too dense to realize it deserve to die bachelors. (And ladies, accept nothing less. Remember what Louise told Thelma, *"You get what you settle for."*) As C.S. Lewis so poignantly put it:

> *In a sort of ghastly simplicity we remove the organ and demand the function. We make men without chests and expect of them virtue and enterprise.* **We laugh at honor and are shocked to find traitors in our midst.**

The Day of America is gone--for now.

Men without chests. Children without morals. And women who put up with both. A country without honor, probably without a future. And we've allowed it to happen. Thinking it cute to fingerpaint with a turd, we're now drowning in a cesspool--a cosmic payback if I've ever seen one. America was a brilliant rocket of a nation which launched from a wilderness and illuminated the globe with a colorful explosion of accomplishment. She's now falling to earth, just a fizzle of smoking ashes and cardboard.

The show's over, the enchantment gone, and the world is laughing. Not politely snickering, but *laughing*. We are fat and soft and whining and stupid, and everyone knows it but *us*.

Our modern savagery

The concomitant blood sports are just arriving (i.e., *The Ultimate Fighting Championship*). Read *The Report from Iron Mountain* and its proposed revival of brutal sports to quench the mass blood lust.

"Now how much would you pay? But, wait! Don't answer!" America is right on the verge of a savage race war. The inner cities have become sprawling factories of thugs meaner than July rattlesnakes, but without their morals. Acoustic flatulence oozes from every stereo, incessantly urging teenage *gangstas* to *"kill that pig."*

To understand just how far we've regressed, watch one of the 1950's grade-school "Mr. Courteous" films where, *"Thomas knows to say 'Please' and 'Thank you!' and to wait his turn in line."* Or, watch any episoide of *Dragnet*, whose toughest criminal laughably seems today a wimp. (I remember one show which, in utter seriousness, dramatized the shoplifting of 26¢ of gum!) Yeah, the 1950s were repressed, but I'll take their manners and clean-cut faces any day over our modern wolf-packs of teenagers with the immorality to blush a sailor. And now we're truly *befuddled* at 9 year olds dousing their sleeping parents with gasoline, or crack-house first-graders shooting their classmates? *"How can such things possibly happen?"*

The Patriot Movement

Oh, so you *believe* the Patriot Movement will save America? Larded with New Age opportunists, magicians, dolts, high-pressure profiteers, and phony "Christians,"--not to mention being heavily infiltrated by the feds--*I don't think so.*

People who can neither spell nor correctly use grammar are suddenly legal "experts." The grossly plagiaristic Lynne Meredith can't even properly use, after first forgetting it entirely, a possessive apostrophe in her jumbled book's own *title*. (To be correct, it should be either *Vultures in Eagles' Clothing*, or *A Vulture In An Eagle's Clothing*--but not *Vultures in Eagle's Clothing*. Oh well, your untax dollars at work...)

Another "Patrioteer" (a former cassette tape hypnotist) recently urged going to the Mayan calender because the Gregorian calender is *"out of harmony with the rhythm of the Universe."* (Gee, what's *next*--"I-Cannot-Tell-A-Lie" crystal balls signed by George Washington?) **These are the kind of people we should *trust* to explain court cases and the tax code?**

Expect circus acrobats and fire-eaters any day now... We need more Howard Freemans, not New Age carnies promoting their cheesy *Cliff's Notes* reports on other authors' work.

Truly, if I hear another cheerleader for the Montana Freemen tell me how legally correct and precise they were, but for the mean, old government--I'm gonna hurl. (Anybody so enamored with the common-law lien M.O. scheme should exchange *their* house and car for some Freemen-style paper, and put their money where their mouth is.) Folks, it's bad enough that our monetary system is based on outright fraud and is in the deathgrip of a corporate monopoly, but what we *don't* need is fraudulent currency from ostensible Patriots out to prove a point under the U.C.C. Had they deposited their M.O.'s with Chase Manhattan and then withdrawn FRN's, *that* would have been cute. Swindling car dealerships and hardware stores, however, is absolutely reprehensible.

Though full of quality people, the Patriot Movement has curdled badly since 1994 and is now very *ill*.

What it needs is a healthy dose of *real-world practicality*, not the self-righteous, self-gratifying intellectual masturbation of endless legal study. **The law is becoming increasingly *irrelevant*.** And I do mean *all* law: common, statutory, equity, constitutional and maritime. As so wisely observed by Patrick Henry, petitions and legal supplications have never forced a committed, oppressive government to set free the people. My friend Linda Sanders, came to the same conclusion and admitted it in her courageous open letter of 5 June 1996:

> *I have been in court--constantly for the past 3 years. I have presented the evidence that has circulated through the Patriot movement--including Karl Granse's regulation argument, Richard*

> *MacDonald's Citizenship argument, Mitch Modeleski's jurisdiction argument, David Myrland's 83(a) argument, Wayne Bentsen's IMF argument and my own Statutes at Large argument. Most of them were proven accurate, by virtue of the Court's (sic) conspicuous omission of a rebuttal.*
> **Did any of them win?**
> *The closest we ever get to a "win" is a suspension of collection--which means the victim's paycheck and house is safe--UNTIL the court decides to do what all courts eventually do--commit treason and rule against Truth, Fact and Law.* **There are no guarantees as to when that will happen.** *I admit that some of my friends are still in "suspension" and have "victories" for about 2 years or less. BUT--I do not boast about this--**because the judicial system is arbitrary and capricious and could render an adverse decision any time they feel like it**--which would give the local sheriffs a reason to practice a swat team raid against those "bad Constitutionalists."*
> *...That does not necessarily mean the research is defective--it means that the courts just won't recognize it.*

Even my own recent book, *You & The Police!*, has a narrowing window of opportunity. Get it and use it while you *can*. Soon, the entire Supreme Court will pack up and go home, leaving a note for Congress and the President saying, *"Do whatever you think is fair. We trust you! XOX, The Justices."*

The law no longer works because America has spun off her legal axis. We are entering the classic final stages of a civilization's cycle. To work, the law requires a decent society made up of literate, responsible individuals who respect the property rights of others. **That society no longer exists.** Today, nearly *half* the country gets a government check, and nearly half of *them* cannot read. **Relying on the law today is like relying on iodine to stop gangrene.** It's too late for topical remedies and we're too wimpy to cut off the leg. Apparently, we'll go down with the putrefying, black stump of our "Land of the Free, Home of the Brave" Mythology. **Freedom requires bravery.** We'll rather die clutching our illusions than bravely face the truth. Oh, well. Every nation since past went through the same thing. We merely completed the cycle at our typical blur.

> *America is the only nation in history which miraculously has gone directly from barbarism to degeneration without the usual interval of civilization.*
> -- Georges Clemenceau (1841-1929)

Just so. Here ends the venting. Thanks for your patience.

So, what's my *point?*

We're now entering a new era in the struggle for Liberty. Parroting U.C.C. 1-207 and state Citizenship arguments won't cut it. It *might* have, thirty years ago. (I wrote *Good-Bye April 15th!* in the good faith hope that a quality legal approach would crack the IRS fraud wide open. Sadly, it's too *late* for that.) **What's become important is what actually *works.***

So what does this all have to do with *privacy?* I'll *tell* you what: **privacy *works.*** Privacy means *insulation* from our curdling society. It means a respite from the growing insanity of our culture. Those of you who want to be grist for the New World Order mill, go right ahead. Give this book to somebody else, and save yourself the read. But to those of a less sacrificial bent, use *this* book while you *can.* **Privacy *works.***

In case you've been asleep in a salt mine since 1968-- the world has gone *nuts.* While I can't change that, I can at least carve out a peaceful oasis for myself and the family I hope to someday raise. I will not move to the rhythm of insignificant others. I want only to be left alone by the mob.

I see no compelling reason why *any* individual should have his domicile vulnerable to strangers or officials. Naturally, I want chosen family and friends to be able to phone me and drop by, but to the rest of the world I am like a ghost. *I* decide who knows where I live and who can call me.

Throughout my years, I've experimented with and lived the life of privacy. Not secrecy, but quality solitude. After much deliberation, I've decided to share many (though not all) of my techniques with you. What I've learned works, and works *well.*

Since *anyone* can be found with enough time and effort (*e.g.,* Eichmann), or reward money (*e.g.,* Gordon Kahl), the trick is remaining not *worth* significant time, effort or reward money.

I sincerely hope that *Bulletproof Privacy* is helpful to you and many thousands like us. Batten down the hatches, a real storm is coming! I will not run, but I will *hide.*

*Our aim is nothing less than to create a world system of financial control in private hands to dominate the political system of each country and the world economy as a whole. **Freedom and choice will be controlled within very narrow alternatives by the fact that** [every man] **will be numbered from birth, and followed, as a number,** through his educational training, his required military or*

other public service, his tax contributions (sic), *his health and medical requirements, and his final retirement and death benefits.*
  -- Carroll Quigley; *Tragedy and Hope* (1966)

As a teenager, I heard John Kennedy's summons to citizenship. And then, as a [draft-dodging] *student at Georgetown, I heard that call clarified **by a professor I had named Carroll Quigley.***
  -- Bill Clinton, accepting the Democratic nomination, on 16 July 1992

Let no more be heard about the New World Order being a paranoid myth of the Patriot Movement. The NWO has been a coordinated, energetic plan for decades. So confident were the Insiders in *1933* (with the election of their man, FDR), that they bragged about it on the Ø1 bill--*"Annuit Coeptis Novus Ordo Seclorum"*--Announcing the Birth of the New World Order. These words frame a 13-level Masonic pyramid with the capstone Eye of Lucifer, just in case anybody needed a symbolic hint.

Here comes our Brave New World--from *Microsoft!*
  The overriding obsession of Bill Gates is biotechnology--how genetic code is similar to binary code, how in the future humans would be downloaded onto chips, and the human spirit burned into silicon to replace the carbon-based host:

> *The most interesting thing to me is not sequencing the data.* **It's understanding the [genetic] *program.*** *How does it work?*
> **Well, someday they're gonna unravel this** (DNA code) **and we'll actually be able to put people onto chips. And the rest is a software** (control of the hardware) **problem.**
>   -- Stephen Manes and Paul Andrews; *Gates*, p.456

We're in for control measures that will make Nazi Germany look pastoral. We're in for a vicious persecution of *anybody* unaccepting of that control: Libertarians, Christians, noncentrist Republicans and Democrats, to name a few.

> **If you want a picture of the future, imagine a boot stamping on a human face--forever.**
>   -- George Orwell; *1984*

Go private, folks--while you *can.* Yeah, all this sounds "alarmist", but don't scoff at volcanos just because lava isn't running all over your feet right now. Go *private.* You can always revert if it turns out that I was out of my mind... *Ciao!*

HOW TO MESS UP

An adventure is usually the penalty for lousy planning.
-- Shorty Jenkins, miner & prospector, 1943

Let me show you how poor privacy techniques will work *against* you. In *The Manhunter*, U.S. Marshal fugitive catcher John Pascucci outlined how he caught the escaped Nazi war criminal Bodhan Koziy from an original nine month time line (the amount of lead time a wanted person has on his pursuers).

First, Koziy mentioned to various neighbors that he was going to Albuquerque or Toronto or Costa Rica. His neighbors also told Pascucci that Koziy had sold his fridge, which meant that he'd probably left (at least) the state. Calling the newspaper, Pascucci traced the 12 September classified ad. He then called every moving company and found the one which had moved the Koziys on the 20th. Talking to a mover, he learned that the stuff went to a warehouse for a couple of days and then was shipped to Albuquerque. Koziy's son lived there.

The son was totally uncooperative. Yes, he knew where his dad was, but he wasn't talking. (Since Koziy was wanted only for a civil matter, his son couldn't be compelled to talk.)

Pascucci then leaned on a Jewish surnamed exec at American Express to get Koziy's charge records. Scanning the sheets for "triggers" (pieces of info which lead to even more pertinent pieces) he noticed a travel agency charge. Plane tickets had been purchased to Albuquerque, Toronto, and Costa Rica. A Waldenbooks charge was quickly identified as *Fodor's Guide to Costa Rica.* But even this didn't break the case:

I know that for fictional detectives, A leads to B, which leads to C, and breaks the case. But in real life, A leads to B, which leads to

> *dick, and then the information that breaks the case waltzes in from left field.*
>
> *But that's not because of luck; it's because you're working in several directions at once.*

Koziy's "driver's abstract" (a DMV record more detailed than the standard profile) said that he'd been in a minor traffic accident with a G. Morelli, which turned out to be his married daughter. Pascucci weaseled Gina's phone records from S.E. Bell, which showed three calls to Costa Rica. He flew there.

The calls had been made to pay phones in lobbies of three different San José hotels. In one of the hotels, Pascucci noticed a car rental agency and learned that Koziy had rented a car, driven it for 90 km. and returned it on 16 April. The time line had shrunk to less than a month, and Koziy was probably living within a 45 km. radius.

A routine airport surveillance photo of incoming nonresidents confirmed that Koziy *was* in Costa Rica. An old address of Koziy's was found, but he had moved 15 days prior. In that time 120 new phone lines had been connected, 95 of which were residences.

Pascucci then had a real-time record of Gina's calls started. Once accomplished, a U.S. Marshal visited her with a sham "no prosecution" deal for her father. As predicted, she immediately called Costa Rica, and the number was one of the new 95 residential numbers. From there, it was easy.

Learning from a Nazi's mistakes

The lesson in all this is that even a very *light* trail leading to you will work as well for an investigator as a very heavy trail. A trail is a trail, and good investigators will pick up the light trails. **Leave no trail whatsoever.** Besides being a creep who wiped out dozens of Jewish families, Koziy's mistakes were:

❶ **Mentioning to *anyone* his destination of Costa Rica.**
His first basic mistake. It made Pascucci think internationally. The Toronto misinfo was great, and Albuquerque was credible as his son lived there, but mentioning Costa Rica blew it.

❷ **Selling his stuff from his *own* place.**
He should have taken it directly to a buyer, or had his daughter sell it for him later. The neighbors shouldn't have known of its disposition so they couldn't have then updated the time line.

❸ Placing a classified ad in his *own* name and number.
Plain stupid, unless done for misinfo. He could have gotten a
temporary voice mail number posing as somebody just briefly in
town. The ad clarified the time line enough for Pascucci to
phone all the movers with a general date of Koziy's move.

❹ Having a listed mover transport his stuff.
Really stupid. He should have moved it himself, or with the
help of some college kids--off the record. Use *bona fide* movers
only for misinfo. At least move your stuff to another city, and
have the mover pick it up from there to break up the trail.

❺ His son *admitting* that he knew where his dad was.
There was *no* reason to admit this. His son should have
expressed strong dislike for his father. Although this mistake
didn't materially help Pascucci, it *could* have.

❻ Charging travel-related items on a credit card.
Unbelievably stupid. Use your credit card *only* for utterly
neutral and bland charges, or for misinformation. Besides one's
phone records, credit card charges are the biggest triggers.

❼ His daughter making calls from *her* phone to Costa Rica.
Catastrophically stupid. It broke the case. He should have
called *her*. It is *far* more difficult to trace the *origin* of an
international call, especially long after the fact.

❽ Renting a car in a the same hotel where he was called.
An easy error to make. If you're receiving a call somewhere,
make sure that no person or camera is around to identify you.
Also, *never* transact business nearby, much less in the same
building. Travel good distances to make/receive your calls.

❾ Not having a *2nd* safe house/phone *already* established.
Also an easy error to make. If you think you might have to bolt,
you should set up your next place, phone and vehicle in advance
so that old and new records don't relay to each other.

It may seem like I'm confusing hindsight with wisdom.
**Much of wisdom is using the *hindsight* of others as your
foresight.** Remember, all the mistakes in Life have *already*
been made by the 100 billion dead *before* you. Wisdom actually
consists of *not* reinventing the *square* wheel. Learn from others' mistakes because there is not enough *time* to learn the Lesson from purely your *own* mistakes--that's lesson #1.

That's what my book will show you--not to be *redundantly* **stupid.** You'll probably get found out by some common gaff; you're unlikely to be found out by through some truly unprecedented error.

However, if you *are,* write me so we all can *learn* from it.

❖ 3

THE RULES

To be successfully private requires the observance of several crucial rules. Extrapolate from these, and you'll do fine.

Don't draw attention to yourself.

Don't be overtly covert. Privacy is about being covertly overt--*seeming* like normal folks at the surface level. If you behave mysteriously or suspiciously, you've already lost, in the long run, your *war* for privacy. The general public and the government shouldn't have any idea that you're a private person, because they'll resent you for it.

Privacy is always *complicated*. Think it through. Avoid crossovers with a schematic.

Even the most *basic* privacy stance (without the use of aliases and ID) is still fairly complicated. For example, you wouldn't want the bill from your secret voice mail sent to the mailing address reserved for government and generic commercial correspondence.

Therefore, you must draw out the linkages of who-knows-what with an electronic-style schematic. You simply will *not* be able to conjure and manage all this in your mind--*trust me on this*. Without a schematic you'll miss some hidden crossovers, and if you're ever *really* scrutinized, the investigator will most assuredly draw out a schematic and discover them.

Privacy is *expensive*. Don't be greedy.

I have a friend who is wonderfully prepared to ditch his city life and relocate to his well-stocked farm retreat three hours away. Having visited his retreat, I'm almost envious. Set on 50 acres in a quiet valley, he's got food (stored and growing), a small cabin, spare vehicles, fuel, and all the supplies he and his wife are likely to need. He's cultivated good relations with his neighbors and is already trading with them to mutual advantage. In a word, he's *set*. At the drop of any ominous hat (martial law, economic collapse, etc.), he's there.

One small problem: he's already *blown* his privacy. How? Not by arranging the property purchase over his home phone (unless his line was monitored). No, what blew his privacy (and he's yet to appreciate this) is that he operates his "Omega Man" retreat as a commercial farm--*and declares it on his tax forms!* By wanting that tax deduction, *by loving the money more than the privacy*, his retreat is all for naught. If the feds ever become interested in him, all they'll have to do is simply pull up his 1040's. He might as well have gotten a listed phone number.

Privacy is expensive. Even the most basic stance will cost about Ø40 per month. **Don't be greedy.** Recognize the costs (emotional, social, and financial) and pay them without grousing about it. Don't try privacy if it's too costly, because you'll get cheap on yourself and ruin the whole game.

Privacy is *inconvenient.* Don't be lazy.

The best laid-out plan with all the expensive frills can be-- no, *will* be--devastated by just *one* lazy slip. *Laziness* will be most tempting in the use of telephones. It's highly inconvenient to have to leave your house to make an alias pay phone call across town. (This is why I strongly discourage your having a home phone. It's just too *easy* to misuse.) Yet if you succumb to laziness that *one* time, and your line has a pen register or trap, that one phone call *will* unravel your tightly wrapped scheme.

Just *one* good loose end is *all* an investigator needs. **Loose ends are created by poor planning and lazy tradecraft.** I've read several hundred true-crime accounts and detective novels to understand this well. In an multi-million dollar insurance fraud, the allegedly deceased husband (from a small plane crash in the ocean) kept in touch with his wife by calling her at the same pay phone at the same time. His supposed death was brilliantly planned and executed. He went to ground without error. Calling *her* was clever (no long-distance records on her line), but using the *same* pay phone was *lazy*. The PI, having followed her, became suspicious since it's not normal to be called *at* a pay phone. He simply bugged the pay phone, and discovered his location in San Juan. Had they used *several* pay phones, they would have pulled it off.

Privacy is *private*. Don't be glib.

A convicted drug dealer posted a Ø1,000,000 pre-sentencing bond and bolted with his wife and children. Having planned his run for months, he was in perfect shape to succeed with other Ø1.5M salted away.

His first mistake, after several months, was to contact his family and friends. During a skip trace, if nothing is uncovered within a few weeks, a good investigator will put the case on a shelf for a few months and work on other things. He knows that everyone slips up--if not immediately, then after a few months of being on the run (which is tedious and nerve-racking). So, after a few months, he began to miss his family and friends.

Using several mail forwardings in series to hide his location, he wrote his mother and sent pictures of his children. One photo, taken outdoors, clued the feds that he was in Virginia. What clinched it was his bragging in a letter that he, a convicted felon on the run, had befriended a retired FBI agent.

The feds simply wrote to all Virginia-area retired FBI agents. The befriended agent read it and, of course, turned in his new buddy. Don't be glib.

Be *consistent*. Be *thorough*.

If bulletproof privacy is important to you, then think it through ahead of time, be consistent, and fight the urge of convenience. ***Nothing else will do*--trust me on this.** Privacy measures add up to a *life-style* which rewards you with the tranquility you've dreamed about. The privacy life-style is an indispensable *means* to that end. **You cannot enjoy *that* end without *those* means.** Know this in advance and make a quality commitment. Don't fool yourself into thinking half-assed measures will accomplish your goals. They *won't*. As Hans and Franz would say, *"Believe me now, or hear me later."*

Work your story out in advance.

Don't allow yourself to be surprised. Know beforehand what is required of a transaction and be prepared for it. Don't be too pat with your recitation, however. Yarns are *weaved*.

Always have a benign, logical explanation.

When asked for your phone number, reply that it's unlisted, or that you've just moved and haven't had one connected yet, or that you're staying with friends and can't give out their number, or that you're just passing through town.

Privacy requires the spinning of yarns.

Though, I'll discuss this more fully in its own chapter, know in advance that you will most likely have to "lie." Would you tell a mugger about your money belt, or would you "lie"? Similarly, our system and society is bent on stealing your quiet joy. You will have to "lie" to protect your privacy.

Be friendly. Be relaxed. Be unremembered.

Surly people are not only remembered--they're *talked about*. *"This guy came in today--geez, what an *sshole!"* The *last* thing you want is to be talked about. Keep your cool and avoid making poor impressions.

Nervous behavior will strike people as odd. It makes them curious, if not outright suspicious. Nervousness is quenched by confidence--confidence is gained by success--success comes from experience, and experience comes from, well, *experience*. This isn't armchair stuff. You'll have to actually go out and *do* it. After a while, it'll be second nature.

Privacy requires your alertness.

This is especially true if you're due for any official scrutiny. You must develop sensitive antennae and keep them up at all times. Before being moved on, you *will* have *some* advance warning: frequent airplane overflights, vehicle drive-bys, a noticeable change in the attitude of bank and postal clerks, a sudden increase in hang up calls, new acquaintances who ask too many questions or too readily agree with your views, your friends and family being quietly sniffed out, etc.

You will have warning signs. In *The Silent Brotherhood*, FBI agents were often spooking their neo-Nazi targets (who usually lost their tail, and even escaped capture on several dramatic occasions). Had the suspected Unabomber not been *so* successful a hermit, he'd have heard about the swarm of feds in Suburbans milling about his lonely county for weeks. (Understand that I've no sympathy with "The Order" and the Unabomber is a malignant coward. I'm simply sharing an observation from their cases.)

Stay alert and you'll probably avoid being surprised. **Alertness, however, is *not* paranoia.** Paranoia is a mental disorder of delusional grandeur and persecution so acute as to be paralyzing. You probably aren't so grand as to be so persecuted--so don't whip yourself into a frenzy. Do as much as you can for yourself, relax and try to *enjoy* life.

❖ 4

PRIVACY & DATA

THE DATA TRAIL

You go through life dropping little bits of data about yourself everywhere. Following right after are big vacuum cleaners sucking them up. -- Evan Hendricks, editor of *Privacy Times*

Computer databanks are awesome, but they're also vulnerable. They rely on *input* and are therefore *lazy*. You can use the system against itself to create a false confidence. If you insist that utterly *no* records exist on you, then you'll quickly attract the attention of some flesh-and-blood investigators, as a blank file is highly unusual and suspicious. So, have a fat file, but *you* are the one who feeds it with good-looking, dead-end data.

Credit information

The Ø800+ million credit reporting industry is dominated by the Big Three: TRW, Equifax, and Trans Union. Other than the feds themselves, these companies are the largest repositories of information about us--nearly 450 million files on 160 million people. Just about anybody with an allegedly relevant business purpose can learn your credit transactions, SSN's, birthdates, mortgage records, employment and salary histories, telephone numbers (even if nonpublished), and information on legal matters, family makeup, bankruptcies, tax liens and your current as well as previous addresses.

The comforting side to all this is that *you* are usually responsible for disclosing all this data--they get it passively. Thus, *you* can misinfo the system to your desire, and it will be reported as fact. With my help, a mail drop will show as your physical address and a voice mail as your telephone number-- not to mention other diversions. Relax.

Employment Information Service (EIS)

If you've ever filed for workman's compensation or sued an employer, you're likely to be blacklisted by this Gretna, Louisiana databank.   Founded in 1966 as a nonprofit corporation by oil and gas bigwigs (including George Bush's Zapata Oil), it maintains nearly a million files.

Then, there are databankers specializing in pre-employment criminal background checks, such as the Information Resource Service Company (IRSC) which tells whether a person has been arrested--even if no conviction resulted.

Medical Information Bureau (MIB)

This non-government databank contains summaries of health conditions on more than 12,000,000 Americans and Canadians (who regularly flee their own socialized health care). The data comes from insurance applications, physicians' files and hospital records. Hospital gossip and miskeyed entries end up as file "gospel" which is nearly impossible to retort or remove. The MIB distributes nearly 30,000,000 reports a year. These files are not all private.   Clerks, salesmen and investigators access them regularly.

Once the federal Human Genome Project is complete, nobody with "defective" genes will likely qualify for health insurance. We're on the brink of a vast, computerized eugenics program envious of Nazi concentration camp "doctors."

Government databanks

I won't exhaustively list them all, but here are the biggies.

National Crime Information Computer (NCIC)

*It's a fast-moving brokerage of criminal data over which information is exchanged by **sixty-four thousand** law enforcement agencies throughout the United States and Canada. NCIC responds to more than one million inquiries every day, or about 11.5 per second. Currently there's only raw computerized data available on NCIC. But soon police will be able to download into their NCIC terminals, many of which are in squad cars, fingerprints, photos, and descriptions of other physical attributes, such as tattoos,...*

If NCIC only bartered in records of convicted criminals, it would be hard to complain about... **But NCIC goes much deeper.** *...[I]t also supplies files on individuals in trouble (whatever* that *is) with local authorities for any number or reasons: people arrested but not convicted of crimes, people with radical (whatever* that *is) political leanings, and people whom law enforcement authorities consider worth watching more closely because they're suspected of real crimes* **or because their behavior is erratic or eccentric.**
   -- Jeffrey Rothfeder; *Privacy For Sale,* (1992) p.130

Even *this* isn't "good" enough; the FBI wants to reshape and expand it to "NCIC 2000" with free, unquestioned access to databanks at airline reservation systems, car rental companies, banks, retailers, credit bureaus, insurance and phone com-pa-nies--not to mention IRS, SSA and INS records. Never mind that current NCIC records are woefully inaccurate and stale.

On a chilling note, the FBI has been spending Ø2 *billion* annually since 1988 to create a national DNA databank. Ostensibly for only known offenders, parents of missing children and individuals who cannot be positively identified, this will eventually extend to all Americans. (The feds would like all newborns to get a heel stick before leaving the hospital.)

Treasury Enforcement Communications System (TECS II)
   Located in Newington, Virginia, TECS II determines if somebody entering the U.S.A. has committed previous customs violations or is wanted by other government agencies. When you and/or your license plate number is entered at one of nearly 300 ports of entry, the system searches through 100 million of its own records, plus those of the DEA, FBI and the DoD. Any person flagged will be at least detained.

   When newsletter author and speaker Don McAlvany entered Denver with his family, the customs agent knew infor-mation extremely varied and detailed--including which hospital his son was born in! I'd get your international travelling done with quickly, before the system becomes even more intrusive.

   Worse than its quasi-omniscience is its gross *inaccuracy.* A secret 1990 study by the GAO found errors in **59%** of the sampled records. This means dirtbags can enter undetected while you and I are erroneously detained and inspected.

Financial Crimes Enforcement Network (FinCEN)

This is the Treasury Department's sophisticated network using "artificial intelligence" to investigate complex financial dealings among disparate individuals and institutions. FinCEN has 200 employees from the IRS, FBI, Secret Service and the FDIC and works closely with the BATF, NSA, INS, FDIC, DEA, CIA and DIA. It can access over 135 financial databases, including land and real estate records, and credit reports.

Created in 1990 ostensibly to catch drug-related money-laundering operations, FinCEN was *really* formed to to centralize financial information on honest Americans. According to Congressman Ron Paul, the feds admit that FinCEN is a trial run for a world system and they also admit that they want all bank employees to function as spies for the government. Its director bragged that FinCEN *"is a lot like Big Brother."*

FinCEN heavily relies upon Forms 4789 (Currency Transaction Report, or CTR's) and 8300 (the retailers' equivalent). More on all this in the chapter *Your Financial Privacy*.

Your state's DMV and vehicle registration

Again, they only know what you *tell* them. It's plain foolish to register your car in your own name and address-- especially if you're an attractive single woman. At the minimum, form a private trust (or Nevada or Wyoming corporation) with a P.O. box address to own your public assets.

In Chapter 13 I'll show you how to create a seemingly valid *street* address which is completely bogus. Such serves as your "official" address for all licensing and registration.

PAPERS

This is simple advice: If you don't *absolutely* need it, don't keep it! The paper trail is like a wake for others to follow. For example, I do not keep handwriting samples, travel schedules, non-vital receipts, routine letters, magazine labels, old gun catalogs, previous working drafts of my writing, etc.

And how do I "not keep" them? Only one method of disposal meets my standard: burning. You should thoroughly burn the bits of your own paper trail at *least* monthly, if not weekly. Leave a short wake behind you. You'd be amazed at how many people have been arrested and convicted by evidence found in their trash. Don't throw it away, *burn* it! Soak the ashes, too. For you recycling mavens, how much is the reusable value worth compared to your privacy?

For those of you still paying income taxes, store your receipts and diskettes *away* from your house or business. These records should be available only at *your* disposal, not the IRS. during some raid (which happens more often than you'd think).

Never carry around with you revealing paperwork. (I cover this in my *You & The Police!*) Right now, go through your own wallet or purse and imagine what all those bits of paper would tell about you to a complete stranger. Would your home address or phone number be found? A sensitive "To-Do" list? Travel plans? Private correspondence?

If you must *temporarily* have such paperwork with you on the road, then keep it in a combination-lock briefcase in the trunk. This offers a firm, legal barrier to all general searches.

PRIVACY & YOUR COMPUTER

I am not a computer expert, as I only use them incidentally for work. Therefore, if you're *seriously* into hard-core computer privacy and data-encryption, you'll need to do some personal research. **You *must* get these two books:** *The Underground Guide to Computer Security* by Michael Alexander (ISBN 0-201-48918-X) and *Data Security* by Janet Endrijonas (ISBN 1-55958-750-4).

Thou shall *encrypt* thy data

All data is illuminating, if not incriminating. Many Patriot groups have been raided by the feds, without arrest. The feds "only" took their computers and diskettes. They do this to learn of an organization's network.

Therefore, I strongly urge not keeping *any* plaintext data on your hard disk. It must be encrypted, through either the IDEA or RSA algorithm. The government doesn't use DES for classified material--which speaks volumes. IDEA (privately developed in Europe) is stronger than even Triple-DES.

There is encryption software (i.e., PGP, or RSA Secure) and hardware (PC cards which I mention in 11/6-7). Send off for information immediately and install something quickly--

especially if you use a laptop. For your password phrase, pick out something obscure yet memorable.

Know this: *any* encryption algorithm can be broken *given sufficient time and resources.* However, your data is not likely worth the NSA spending 500 years of computer time to crack-- and *that's* what makes encryption practical.

PRIVACY & TECHNOLOGY

*Soon it will be possible to assert almost continuous surveillance over every citizen and maintain up-to-date complete files containing even the most personal information about citizens. **These files will be subject to instantaneous retrieval by the authorities.***
-- Zbigniew Brezhinsky; *Between Two Ages*

Databanks are manifestations of computer technology. But what *is* technology? It is merely the multiplication of human effort by artificial means. It is not magic, it is only *leverage.* As leverage, it multiplies the *effect and scope* of the operator.

Technology is vital to oppressive governments as they simply *cannot afford* man-on-man surveillance. East Germany tried it and went bankrupt. In Romania, one citizen in *five* was a paid government informant. (Romania never *went* bankrupt--it never *escaped* bankruptcy.)

Governments rely upon technological leverage to be quasi-omnipresent, and omnipresence is the prerequisite to omnipotence. **Any leverage, however, requires a *fulcrum.* That fulcrum is *knowing on whom to focus.*** By being a *public* agitator, you've given government the necessary fulcrum to use its techno-leverage against you. Neutralize that fulcrum and the lever itself is rendered useless. By being private, we force on government an inefficient, costly and ineffective system of Romanian man-on-man surveillance. The government *cannot* win without its techno-leverage and its broad-based social conditioning through the media megaphones.

While we are working to counter the social conditioning, not enough is being done to counter government's techno-leverage. There are a few ways to do this:

Even the playing field by matching technology.
This is difficult, expensive and time-consuming. Americans simply don't have the required time and money. While we

do need some really well-equipped people, we just can't afford it *systemically.* (However, if you've the money, you can equip yourself *nearly* as well as the black bag boys. Get your long-range rifles, bulletproof vests, encrypted radios, night vision and range-finding gear *now*--while it's still possible.)

The battle between the rulers and the ruled is (for now) primarily one of *information.* For example, the putative collapse of Soviet communism was greatly assisted by the mass influx of computers and fax machines. Similarly, the Federal Government is fast growing panicky over the explosion of talk radio, desktop publishing, digital encryption and the Internet.

Especially the Internet. No wonder the feds are pushing for an "Information Highway" (singular). *One* superhighway would be easiest to control. (They'd rather prohibit the thing altogether, but they're too late. That particular cat is already out of the bag.) What we need, and what we'll probably succeed in getting, are *several* highways and hundreds of smaller roads.

Information, however, is merely *one* key--it is not *the* key to our eventual Liberty. Once governments realize that they've lost the information battle, they'll see no choice but to resort to the blackmail of *food.* Hungry people, regardless of their informational capabilities, will "see the light":

> *Food is power. We use it to change behavior. Some may call that bribery. We do not apologize.*
> -- Catherine Bertini, Exec. Dir. U.N. World Food Program
> U.N. 4th World Conference on Women, Sept. 1995

We're winning the information battle, but at the same time let's also enhance our physical self-sufficiency and preparedness. Move to the country, till the soil, homeschool your children and train with the firearms you *should* have by now *already* acquired. The communication privacy measures I outline *are* important, but do not ignore the *physical* measures.

Low-cost countermeasures

A private life is an example of this. The NVA's method of warfare against us in Vietnam is another. **Remember, the finer the net, the more *slowly* it must be trolled.** As long as you remain a bright, quick, little fish--the net won't catch you. Sure, the net *will* catch millions of human shrimp, but you and I will not be one of them.

We *want* government to stay top-heavy and rely mostly upon its expensive techno-leverage. We want them to be vulnerable to the weather, quirky satellites, and an unexpected shortage of AA cell batteries. Folks, night vision devices and laser range-finding gear is neat stuff, but first learn to live and fight without it. Never rely upon the "gravy."

Rendering oppressive technology moot

Technology has always been a double-edged sword, and a fairly neutral one at that. Who gets cut by it largely depends upon who wields it from the *higher* position. If you can't gain elevation on your opponent because he controls the high ground, don't just stand there. **Leave the room and make his sword irrelevant.** The government is stronger and taller than us. Did David slog it out with Goliath? No. David kept his distance and calmly put a rock in Goliath's temple. He made Goliath's strength and height *irrelevant.*

Similarly, we *cannot* beat the government in a slugging match. But that's O.K.; one should never fight the *enemy's* game--make him fight *yours.* My view is that we should concentrate on using the tools we have *today* to *circumvent* the system and force a paradigm shift. Freedom-loving individuals should have their *own* private CommNet and their *own* economic system (preferably in encrypted digital form backed by warehoused gold). Let the government swat at *air.*

So, FinCEN will have real-time access to our credit card and banking transactions. *So what?* **We'll quit using them in favor of DigiCash.** Try to paint us into a corner and we'll jump to another *building.* Then they'll have to start all over.

Personally and systemically, we need to transform into *ghosts.* This book is about the *personal* transformation. An upcoming book will address the *systemic* transformation, but we'll need many more individual ghosts before our vaporish world can be possible. **We must first neutralize the government's leverage and force to them to go "man-on-man."** *Then* it will be a personal battle which no American can *ignore. Then* it will be the personal battle which no government has ever *won.*

We *can* make the oppressive "real-world" irrelevant. The tyrants first made freedom inconvenient and then out of reach. We will wield that *back* edge of the technological sword.

We will swing that sword and win back our country.

THE VITAL ATTITUDE

"WHAT IF I HAVE TO *LIE?*"

To answer this requires a philosophical aside. First of all, it is not illegal to use an alias *so long as there is no fraudulent intent.* For example, it's pretty obvious that "Boston T. Party" is not my given name. I use this *nom de plum* to afford myself a bit of privacy and to evoke a fun, patriotic flavor. There is no intent to defraud anyone.

Now, let's take the "innocent alias" concept a bit further. Many privacy measures require representations which are un-true. Remember, all of my books are written, not for bonafide criminals, but for peaceable folk who just want to increase their personal freedom. Thieves, con-men, those who initiate violence, etc. *should* be caught and punished. Such crimes are called *mala in se*--"evil in themselves."

However, *mala prohibitum* ("wrongs prohibited," or rules and regulations concerning victimless offenses) are simply degradations of our Liberty. Emerson once said, *"Good men must not obey the laws (rules) too well."* As long as you don't hurt or rip off people--*as long as there is no fraudulent intent*--these techniques can and should be used with a clear conscience.

By "fraud" I mean intentionally deceiving somebody into acting to their detriment. Throughout my many years of privacy living I have *never* defrauded another. I have established many forms of commercial service under some kind of alias, purely for my own privacy. The bills were always paid. **The moral: Do not hurt others.**

THE PUBLIC FACE OF PRIVACY

When in public, *act* like the public. Never draw attention to yourself. At home, you can skulk about all you want, but in public, do not be overtly covert.

This is absolutely vital when you are establishing your voice mail service, buying plane tickets, applying for alias ID, etc. The clerk must feel perfectly comfortable with the transaction. Don't blow it by being nervous, sarcastic, impatient or rude. Be polite, smile and practice an agreeable banter. Such an attitude is *oil* to the transaction. Do not, however, be *too* polite or officious--do not try *too* hard.

Know in advance the documentary requirements for the transaction and have your "legend" well buttressed and rehearsed. Do not be caught off guard, or else you'll probably stammer and ruin the deal. RELAX! To the clerk, you're just another public face. Be fairly cheerful, yet nonchalant.

Do not make a fuss about: the long wait in line, the bureaucratic pointlessness of the thing, and ID or SSN requirements. **You're there to complete the transaction, and so is the clerk. Give her what she needs, and she'll return the favor.** Do what it takes to accomplish your goal. Regarding the SSN, you either don't have one or you don't know it, or give her a fake one (research the proper birthplace 3 digit sequence and have the fake number done on a metal card). Don't start fulminating about the SSN being some Mark of the Beast prequel (even though we all know it that probably *is*).

Once you've got your paperwork, ID, tickets, etc. you should politely and smoothly bid the clerk a "good day" and leave. Don't gush relief at the counter--have your party later.

It just takes a bit of practice. The first few times you'll understandably be nervous. That's why you should start with the small stuff first (voice mail service, a P.O. box, etc.). Then, when it comes time for bigger transactions, you'll be ready.

❖ 6

PRIVACY & PEOPLE

We live in a human world. While no man is an island, and I wouldn't want to be an utter hermit, being a peninsula suits *me* just fine. Although everybody needs people, a minor link to humanity is enough for me. I prefer to define that link's quality and quantity as much as *reasonably* possible. By itself, such is a weighty task, but when one adds stringent privacy measures the task can become quite formidable.

Since we do live in a human world, you must at least occasionally rub elbows with people. To do so, yet retain privacy, requires a certain kind of person; one who plans ahead, thinks quickly on his feet, has the easy capability to spin yarns, and a *good memory*. Above all, one must have a good memory.

LEVELS OF INTIMACY

You should have concentric levels of trust. The better you know somebody, the more intimate you allow them to become.

Americans are notorious for their immediate "friendships" and first-name/arm-on-shoulder relationships. Though I love our sense of easy rapport, it's often at the cost of incredible shallowness and fickleness. Having lived abroad, I prefer the European *time-based* approach to establishing friendships. There, it generally takes at least a *year* to be considered one's friend. In the Germanic countries, when an elder accepts a youth as a friend it's commemorated by the **Du**zenshaft--an evening of drinks whereby the youth is officially invited to call the elder by the informal *Du* instead of the formal *Sie*.

There is no such equivalent rite of passage in America. We've completely erased any former distinction between acquaintances and friends. We've cheapened our friendships, and though as an insular sociological phenomenon it has escaped our *own* notice, foreigners are painfully aware of it. **My fellow Americans, heed this advice:** if you befriend a foreigner, do not voice invitations to write letters or visit your home unless you will damn well *keep* your promise. When a Dutchman hears that he is welcome in your home when visiting Memphis, he is relying upon your word. Put him up without fail. If his visit's timing doesn't mesh, then put him up at a friend's or at a hotel. Make your word mean something.

I have visited the homes of dozens of foreign friends and never once was an invitation extended to me withdrawn when I was due. When a European invites you as a guest, he *means* it and it is a great honor. (Be a *good* guest. Take his family out to a nice dinner, or leave them a nice gift from America.) Americans, on the other hand, invite frivolously and are shocked when Gunter from Stuttgart actually calls. Our country has bad enough of a reputation. Don't sour it further. If you meet a foreigner traveling through your town and you two hit it off, invite him/her to your home, if for nothing but a coffee. Let's undo decades of damage. O.K., enough on that.

Now that you understand the progression of public--acquaintance--friend--good friend--best friend, let's start.

Privacy with the public

The "public" means clerks, passersby and the like. These people need to know very little about you--only enough to accomplish your goal. They're not generally entitled to your voice mail number and P.O. box, unless absolutely necessary (i.e., during a classified ad sale). Be polite, keep your word, do your deal, and leave. If you like somebody in particular, then he gets to become an acquaintance.

Privacy with your acquaintances

An acquaintance is neither fish nor fowl--neither public nor friend. It is a difficult relationship in America. We are by nature a friendly people, and it's only natural that your acquaintances will want to become your friends. This is not necessarily a bad thing (some of your acquaintances *should* become friends), however, the lesson here is *not* to allow the transformation to be *routine*. In my estimation, of all the people one knows by name, 80% should remain merely acquaintances.

Acquaintances are such because of a basic common interest and affinity. Thus, they will usually deserve to have your voice mail number and mail-drop address, but nothing more. Only friends (and perhaps only *good* friends) should know where you live (or your real name if using an alias). Whatever the common interest, let acquaintanceships remain there until you feel *very* comfortable in befriending them.

Do not significantly avail upon your acquaintances, nor allow them to significantly avail upon you. Such is done only amongst *friends*. Do not call him last minute to take you to the airport or use his lawnmower. Never lend to or borrow from an acquaintance.

If the acquaintance comes to realize that you're intentionally stunting the growth of the relationship (and most won't), he can become hurt or even pushy. You must handle this very adroitly. Even though the issue *is* a personal one, you cannot be unfeeling and coarse about it. Explain that you've been badly hurt in the past and that you've grown to prefer taking longer time in making friends. Most folks will be satisfied with this, and will value a future friendship with you all the more. The rest you should quietly drop as acquaintances. Learn earlier, rather than later.

The acquaintance neighbor

Although he's not a friend, he knows: where you live, many of your habits, and who many of your friends are. **He must be *very* carefully managed.** He is in a position to cause you great grief and inconvenience. (Randy Weaver's problems were much exacerbated by his poor relations with a neighbor.)
The main things to avoid cultivating in your neighbors are: *annoyance, curiosity, suspicion and envy.* Do not flaunt your wealth or share your business with them. Do not get into hassles with them. Keep contact to a minimum, though not suspiciously so. Be cheerful, polite, respectful, moderately helpful--this is the cost of living in town and having neighbors. If you're unwilling or unable to pay this modest fee, then buy hundreds of acres in the country.

Befriending a neighbor acquaintance is not recommended. A neighbor friend is like a marriage. Besides, if you move and he is questioned--can you trust him to not divulge your new location? As wonderful as most of my neighbors have been, I personally have preferred *not* to befriend them and thus be free to relocate without trace. That's often been bewildering to them, however, such is a price of privacy.

Privacy and your friends

Every friendship is a sort of secession, even a rebellion. It may be a rebellion of serious thinkers against accepted claptrap or of faddists against accepted good sense; of real artists against popular ugliness or of charlatans against civilized taste; of good men against the badness of society...

Whatever it is, it will be unwelcome to Top People. In each knot of friends, there is a section which fortifies its members against the public opinion of the community in general. Each is therefore a pocket of potential resistance. Men who have real friends are less easy to manage or "get at"; harder for bad authorities to corrupt. Hence, if our masters, by force or by propaganda about "togetherness" or by unobtrusively making privacy impossible, ever succeed in producing a world in which all are companions and none are friends, they will have removed certain dangers, and will also have taken from us what is almost our strongest safeguard against complete servitude.

-- C.S. Lewis; *The Four Loves*

You probably have the same problem that I *used* to have--*too many friends*. A million rhinestones cannot make wealth, but a handful of diamonds do. I was a Rhinestone Baron, wondering why I was continually disappointed with my friends.

I used to make friends the American way--*profusely*. My PDA once contained over 1,100 people. It was ridiculous. I didn't need so many "friends," but what to do? As the waggish quote goes, *"It's easy to make a friend. What's hard is to make a stranger."* Obviously, I couldn't call up 900 people and tell them they've been to demoted to Acquaintance First Class.

So, I allowed a natural attrition based on an important criterion of mine. Those who kept in regular touch with me *by letter* stayed onboard. I wanted to keep those friends who were letter writers, and who would write to me. Generally, the letter-writing friends have been much better friends than the phone-calling ones. There's just something special about writing a letter, and stamping the envelope. Modern email can't compare. Anyway, this has worked for me. My number of friends is now totally manageable and I enjoy *quality* friendships. I am now a *Diamond* Baron.

Best friends

To me, there are friends, good friends, and *best* friends. A *best* friend is one for whom I'd die defending, and vice versa. A *best* friend understands your need for privacy, and could be trusted with just about all of your secrets. This book's measures will largely be moot for best friends. While one can't have too many best friends, they are so rare and so time-consuming in development that I doubt one could make more than one a year. As I'm still a comparatively young man, I don't have many best friends, but they're increasing. In the times ahead, we will desperately need all the best friends we can make. A man ending up with as many as *six* best friends is wealthy beyond words.

Good friends

A *good* friend is an extremely solid person. He knows many, but not all, of your secrets. He knows your real name and where you live. Hopefully, he is enroute to becoming a *best* friend, but this is not always possible or advisable. You'll know if that's the case. Good friends can easily become jealous of your best friends if they sense a dichotomy. Therefore, friends shouldn't know there are *good* friends and good friends shouldn't know there are *best* friends. Tell them when they've *been* "promoted" but don't warn them of any possible upgrades.

Friends

A "mere" friend is one you trust about a third of the way. You constantly test his strength, reliability and discretion. Is he a whiner, a braggart, or a bully? Find out ASAP. Making a new friend is exciting, but keep things toned down. He's much more than an acquaintance, but much less than a best friend. Remember, he's a *candidate* for bigger things.

In general, friends should make up only *20%* of who you know. "Mere" friends will make up 80% of your friends; good friends 18%; best friends 2%. For example, if you know 1,000 people (and most of you do), 800 should be acquaintances, 160 friends, 36 good friends, and only 4 best friends. I'm being silly, of course, but these figures are in the ballpark.

A good timetable is at least a *year* between levels. Acquaintance, year one. Friend, year two. Good friend, year three. *Best* friend, year four. Folks, I'm not kidding about this! Make being your friend *stand* for something. Make them *earn* it. Would you throw a house together in a month and expect it to shelter you in a storm? Friends are roofs over our heads. Take the time to build a *quality* human shelter.

Girlfriends

More guys have unnecessarily confided sensitive matters to their girlfriends, only to their detriment. Many men in prison today are pondering Shakespeare's wisdom, *"Hell hath no fury like a woman scorned."* You never know a woman until you break up with her. If a woman feels mistreated, then all bets are off. For example, both the wife and mistress of Order leader Robert Matthews rolled over to the feds after his death.

Therefore, if she absolutely doesn't *need* to know something, and you're not defrauding her by your silence--*be quiet.* This takes some diligent compartmentalization. That doesn't make it "bad"--that just makes it *real. Nothing personal.*

Relatives

Do not relax your standards with relatives. Just because a random human is your cousin or sister by complete accident of birth, don't divulge your life secrets unless they've gone through the filtering process. I had the misfortune to arrive amongst a rather unusual family. Weird, actually--chock full of soap-opera intriguing and backbiting. Except for a handful, I've nothing to do with them. (Most don't even know where I live, or what I do for a living.) It was tough not to have a quality support mechanism when I was a boy, but it *did* inculcate self-sufficiency and independence. And, I'll never take my *own* family for granted when I have one.

Be very careful about what phone number and address you give to relatives, even to your own parents. Not so much that they'll purposely betray you, but *inadvertently.* One's relatives are much more easily discovered than one's friends. Relatives will absorb the initial questioning and will be watched the longest. Train them well, or leave them out of the loop.

One P.I. told the story about a skip trace who was close to his out-of-state mother. So the P.I. calls his mother, *"Mrs. Jones, this is Dr. Malcolm at Cleveland General Hospital. Your son, Brian, has been in a severe car accident and we need you to fly out and to identify him and sign some papers."* (or something like that). Mrs. Jones, caught totally off-guard and now in a panic, calls her son's number given to her only for emergencies. The P.I. later got her long-distance records. Clever, huh?

Relatives should be trained not to believe every "old friend" or "emergency" call. Have them say only, *"Give me your name and number. If we hear from him, we'll tell him you called."* They should use a prepaid calling card from a pay-phone to reach you, and *never* dial your home from theirs. Analyzing their MUD's is an easy way to find a skip trace.

Your spouse

If you're *contemplating* marriage, accept nothing less than a best friend. If your spouse is not at least a *good* friend, then you've got problems. Ideally, your spouse should be not only *a* best friend, but *the* best friend you have.

If you're *already* married, making a best friend of your spouse should be your Number One earthly priority. Most men are morons, slaving at a job and thinking that their wives get all turned on by the Good Provider thing. Yes, husbands *should* support their families--but families need *more* than that. Men, take *time* to be *with* your wife and children. **Share yourself, not just your paycheck.** Or, you can hear *Cats and the Cradle* over the radio, and cry enroute to the office in your Mercedes, suddenly realizing how empty your entire life became, why your wife is sleeping with the tennis coach and your children never come to visit. Guys, catch a clue.

I know a married couple in the Movement who are physically well-prepared and own many guns. **Trouble is, she most likely won't defend her husband.** She's been so worn down by his caustic manner, that he has very sadly admitted to me that they were ever actually raided, he would be on his *own.* In such a scenario, I think I'd rather be single than risk the wrath of pissed-off "partner."

That aside, back to privacy. You should develop code gestures, words and phrases, mutually plant caches and test each other's privacy measures. You are a *team.* Perform as one.

Your children

They are *yours*, not the State's. The State, however, wants their minds and souls and bodies--so you will have to *fight* to keep them. This will become increasingly difficult, especially if our Senate ratifies the *U.N. Convention on the Rights of The Child.* (Read the November '96 *MIA* for the full story.)

Maintain *perfect* relations with your neighbors, or else some do-gooder will inform "social services" that your children are undernourished, neglected, abused, etc. Once a case file is started, every local bureaucrat will be hypersensitive to anything regarding your family. You might as well move.

Regarding social behavior, your children should be polite and respectful without volunteering information or answering personal questions. Train them to *never* repeat your actual address to anybody, nor discuss family matters. If ever strenuously questioned by authorities, they should know to reply, *"I don't know. You'll have to ask my parents that."*

Do not divulge to them anything that they do not absolutely *need* to know--especially sensitive activities. As with anybody, trust them only as far as you must. They shouldn't be burdened with heavy family secrets, anyway.

How to not register your children

First rule: *never* get them a "Social Security Number." Hospitals will insist on parents filling out the SSN application before mother and baby check out--*absolutely refuse!* For those of you still filing unrequired Form 1040's, an SSN is asked for all claimed dependents--**but you're *not required* to claim *any* dependents**. Keep them off the tax rolls, even if it costs you the tax deduction. Don't put base monetary greed over your children's legal sovereignty.

You might want to home birth with a midwife, for privacy and to avoid getting a "Birth Certificate" which registers your child with the Commerce Department as a *"national resource."* Create your own "Record of Birth" with signed witnesses.

Their minds

Whatever you do, do *not* send them to public schools. The "education" is worse than poor; it is designed to sap their independence and ruin their critical thinking. The State wants "world citizens"--that is, androids with no American allegiance or strong family ties. Send them to a quality *private* school (one which refuses all federal funding and the attached strings).

If a private school is too expensive or unavailable, then consider home-schooling. You can even join local families to pool resources and expertise. Some states allegedly "require" that you register as home-schoolers, but you could easily avoid that by saying that you're just passing through from Mississippi, Virginia or South Carolina (which have repealed compulsory attendance laws). Stay low key.

Their bodies

Be very suspicious of "compulsory" vaccines. Find out (if you can) exactly *what* is in those flu shots, etc.--before subjecting your children to some mystery vaccine. Many people vaccinated for polio in the 1950's have come down with brain cancer, as the vaccine was mixed with SV-40 (Simian Virus-40). Many reputable doctors and medical experts believe that the HIV (which putatively causes AIDS) was purposely created and mixed in Hepatitis-B vaccines given specifically to male homosexuals in NYC, Chicago, St. Louis, L.A. and San Francisco.

I am personally suspicious of fluoridated water. Sodium fluoride is a by-product of making aluminum and is listed as a *poison* by the CDC. (What do you think *rat* poison is made of? Check the label.) Fluoridated water does *nothing* to enhance teeth hardness as claimed and European countries have outlawed it since the 1970's--so what's *really* the point? What do the French and the Swiss know about it that we don't? Drink well water or distilled water.

ON TRUSTING PEOPLE

For example, fully 90% of all FBI arrests are due directly to the *"helpful cooperation"* of neighbors and relatives. Keep your mouth shut. *Never* get chatty with government officials. Don't talk to the State. Only silence *can't* be used against you.

"Trust only if you can, and then only if you have to."

It's the *second* part of this maxim which will protect you, as trusting is easier than qualifying the absolute *necessity* of trusting particularly. Let me express my aphorism another way: If you believe a person trustworthy on an issue, but can *wait* to find out, then wait. From my own experience, I cannot recall a *single* incident where I *should* have trusted, but did not, or waited too long. I can, however, think of dozens of times where I trusted too early (and sometimes *far* too early).

Trust only at the last minute, so to speak. Why trust too early? There's no advantage, and much potential risk. This is true because of immutable human nature: **People are *verbs.*** Fewer than 5 in 100 you'll ever meet are solid, dependable, and thoroughly trustworthy souls.

The other 95% exhibit merely varying *degrees* of reliability, and some of them *seem* totally trustworthy for quite a while, until a real crunch arrives. Take your time to trust.

Putting friendships to the test

I am retrospectively a big believer in this. Something is reliable only if it's been *proven* to be reliable. If you haven't tested your friendships by important (though not utterly crucial) matters, then you've no idea how strong they really are.

I once knew a couple my age for many years who seemed to be high-quality people. We had spent lots of time together and knew each other well. Then, one day, I needed an urgent favor. It was a big favor to me, but a small one to them (which required no risk or expense and only 5 minutes of inconvenience). They hemmed and hawed and finally declined. (I went to another friend, who immediately and cheerfully agreed.) A few days later, they told me that they'd been *"stupid"* and were profoundly sorry, and now would gladly help. I replied that, while I appreciated their change of heart, tests of friendship often come in sudden moments and that I could never trust them as I once had. (To their credit, they took it well.)

Intentional tests

Trust is like a muscle, and it must be at least sporadically exercised. For example, I make a point of occasionally (say, yearly) lending and borrowing small amounts of money. (Such is collected/paid back within days.) A friend who is not good for $50, a friend who cannot be immediately relied upon for $50, is a very weak friend.

A similar kind of test is entrusting a secret. In all of my friends I've confided one interesting item, unique to their ears alone. (None of them are earth-shattering, but they are juicy enough to tempt any gossiper.) Each friend is a vault for a particular secret, and if one of them gets out, I know the source.

Yes, I realize that all this may sound cold and inhuman, but I'd rather learn of any weakness or betrayal earlier (and in a smaller context), rather than later (and in a crucial matter).

THE I.D.

As I mentioned earlier, I won't get into much detail on alias ID's (manufacture or procurement). I recommend that you peruse the alternative book catalogers (Paladin, Loompanics, Eden, Delta, etc.) as the subject of ID's is too great for this book. Besides, good stuff has already been written and I try not to rehash others' material. Barry Reid's *Paper Trip III* will be published by Eden shortly, and I expect it to be a worthy companion of the first two *Paper Trip*'s.

I have personally come up with an ID methodology which, for my limited purposes, works very well. This methodology, however, is fairly uncommon and particular to my situation--so I can't really divulge it. *But*, what I *will* do is discuss ID's in general terms. I will try to at least steer you the right direction.

Alias ID is fairly risky business. You should carefully consider *who* might be looking for you and how *far* they'll go to find you. Don't *under* construct ID for your situation.

There are three kinds of "cooperative" ID: using somebody else's ID; procuring *bona fide* ID through fake paperwork; and manufacturing what *looks* to be *bona fide* ID. The first two are government issued, and the third you "issue" to yourself. Each have their uses and limitations.

USING ANOTHER'S ID

Assuming that you can procure ID from somebody whom you sufficiently resemble, *and* that you don't get him into trouble, this method can temporarily work.

Finding a near "twin" as your "donor"

Good luck. You might luck into an ID left behind at a bar, liquor store or nightclub. When I was younger and more cardable, I saw many guys' ID's taped up near the front door of my favorite liquor store. It would have been no problem to tell the clerk, _"Oh, hey--that's Charlie's driver's license. I see him everyday in class. Do you want me to take it to him?"_ Though I could have become "Charlie" I never tried it. Anyway, this stunt would likely work with most clerks.

Be aware that a lost ID is noted on the state computer when the holder goes to replace it. A _stolen_ ID is listed in the NCIC. Either way, the ID's usefulness is clearly limited. Any significant computer check (accomplished by any cop with a radio) would reveal that you're not "Charlie."

If, however, you kept the use solely at a supporting role, somebody else's ID could be worthwhile.

Not getting anybody into trouble

Don't use the ID for traffic tickets (even if you intend to pay them promptly). Don't use it for credit purposes (even if you intend to pay the monthly bills). Don't use it if you get detained or arrested. Don't use it to procure supplemental ID, especially a passport. Well, gee--what's left?

Basically, you don't want to create conflicting records with the donor which causes some agency to contact him. You might be able to quietly rent a car under his name (paying with cash), get a library card, rent movies, or establish very minimal local credit (which is not entered in his credit report).

Finally, if your donor got into trouble all by himself, "your" alias could be a ticking bomb. Have fun explaining that you're _not_ "Charlie" and were only using his driver's license. Tee, hee.

USING FAKE PAPERWORK

This is the best option for long-term use. You'll encounter most of your risk during application, but once received you'll be fine as long as you keep a fairly low profile. I wouldn't, however, try to then get a security clearance with the NSA. Any serious background check will quickly bring down your tent.

The application

The younger you are, the easier it is to explain why you're only *now* getting your first driver's license, SSN, or passport.

The birth certificate (BC)

The BC (or its equivalent--church birth record, family Bible record, or newspaper announcement) is the father of all ID's, fake or not. Years ago, people successfully simply used the BC of a deceased infant who would have been their age. The feds have pretty much cataloged the nation's death certificates into a database to prevent that method (especially for passports). Don't use the "dead baby" scam.

Being dead and being *declared* dead are two different things. Only when one is declared dead is a death certificate filed. A BC from a person who became missing *without being declared dead* might work--as long as he *stayed* missing. The research to learn of such a person would be difficult, but I offer the idea, nonetheless.

After much thought, I think that the *best* way is to simply *create* your personality and its own BC.

What the government *doesn't* know and *can't* know is the name of everybody who has been *born*. Many people join the "system" for the first time as adults. They could have been sailing around the world or been children of missionaries. Absent conflicting information or firm suspicion, the government must accept that you are who you *say* you are.

Never forget that. All "knowledge" ultimately derives from a foundational *belief.* **For example, do you have *personal, firsthand knowledge* of your own birthday?** No, you can't--you were a newborn infant without a calender. We must all take our parents' word for it. Similarly, if you concoct a totally fictitious personality and present a concocted BC (or equivalent), the government must take *you* at *your* word.

A believable BC and cover story will get you a driver's license. With a driver's license, you can get *everything* else. Eden Press seems to be the most ID oriented of the alternative book sellers, and I would start there. There are even companies which sell blank BC's (and equivalents).

At the desk, applying for it--you big phony

Remember, this is *routine* for the clerk. Keep it that way. Getting a driver's license for the first time at 43 years of age will seem suspicious. The DL is the hardest to get late in life because *everyone* in America learns drives in high school. But relax; once you have your license the hard part is over. SSN's, credit cards and passports are often originally applied for in one's later years. So, what to tell the driver's license clerk?

Moral: have a plausible story to allay her doubts in under 30 words. Anything longer will *sound* like a story. Tell her that you grew up in NYC and never learned how to drive because you took the subway. Tell her that you were blind from childhood until recently when you had the latest laser surgery. Make it short and sweet, where she goes, *"Oh!"*

You should also have any necessary supporting documentation, such as NYC paperwork (letters addressed to you, club memberships, etc.) or a newspaper article on the miraculous eye surgery you had. Don't make it obvious that you're trying to prove your case. Don't try *too* hard, because that's not routine for applicants.

For your address, *never, never* give your real address. Don't even give out a *friend's* address, however willing he seems to cover for you. (People are *verbs*, not nouns. He would probably roll over on you with enough carrot or stick.)

If the clerk asks for your phone number, reply that you've only been in town for a couple of weeks and that you can't afford it until next month. (Most clerks will silently gloat at their higher monetary status and feel superior to you. That's fine.)

If the clerk seems hinky about the whole thing and excuses herself to *"check on something"*--calmly and politely leave (*"While you're doing that, I'll go get my money. It's in my friend's car."*) Not *your* car, because you don't have a driver's license yet, remember? **Moral: *leave* before chancing an arrest.** You can try again elsewhere under another name.

Using this alias and its ID

So, you fooled them all and got your alias ID. Great, but you're not invincible. Don't get all cocky and think you can get away with anything. Don't piss off some government agency or skip out on your new credit card debt. Don't give anybody *any* reason to start digging in your past--a past which doesn't exist. If you blow this alias, the next one will be harder to create. They'll already be looking for you, and the screening procedure may be tougher (e.g., requiring biometric data) the next time.

TOTAL ID CREATION

Technology is the classic double-edged sword here. Publishing software, color laser printers and high resolution scanners make it possible to create quality documents in your own home. Ragnar Benson's new book, *Acquiring New ID--How to Easily Use the Latest Computer Technology to Drop Out, Start Over, and Get On With Your Life* (ISBN 0-87364-894-3; Paladin Press) covers exactly this. For example, one can literally produce a visually near-perfect driver's license.

The flip side is that government records are well networked by computer and accessible by any diligent cop or fed. There are a myriad of available databases: TECS II (Treasury), EPIC and MIRAC (immigration databanks), NADDIS (the DEA's databank), state DMV's, and the NCIC--to name a few. A fake ID being *visually* persuasive is no longer sufficient; it must now convince the *computers*.

My opinion is that well-crafted ID will work *until* you're subject to some investigation. Most routine computer checks are within databanks listing wanted criminals. Honest folks, clean aliases and extraterrestrials won't be in there. As long as the computer check is simply looking for positive hits and not utter verification of the document and its owner, you should be fine. (Create a totally fake DL from Iowa and the L.A. cop will be real curious why the Iowa DMV has no record of issuing it.) Created ID has its place, but think it through.

The foreign ID

This is undoubtedly the most useful class of created ID. Links to foreign databanks are very slow and spotty. Best of all, nobody here knows what a French DL *looks* like. (When I say "foreign" I mean *really* foreign, not Canada or Mexico.) Don't create French ID unless you can converse fluently in French, because you'll someday encounter a cop who can *parlais*.

When asked to show your U.S. visa, reply that you're only *half* French, that your father is American, and that as a dual national you don't *need* a U.S. visa. This half-and-half story is surprisingly versatile: it explains why you don't have a SSN or state DL. And, as an apparent tourist, you'll be treated with more courtesy and leniency for the small stuff.

Creating it yourself

If you have a foreign friend, ask him to send a photocopy (preferably in color) of his DL and personal ID card. Scan this in your computer and doctor it to your needs.

Be very thorough in your use of foreign materials (paper and staples, which are quite different than domestic supplies). Age your document convincingly with scratches, bent corners and the occasional stain (tea works well).

Have supporting ID in business cards (which are usually oversized), club cards, tram tickets, stamps and currency exchange receipts (your foreign friend can get these for you), etc. **The supporting paper is just as important as the DL.** Read up on the fantastic job the OSS did in WWII for our spies dropped into Axis territory.

Buying foreign ID

A company called RTA (303-727-7962) manufactures Nicaraguan International Driving Permits (IDP's). "Valid" for four years, they cost Ø200. With supporting ID, this might work pretty well, especially if you speak Spanish.

Or, you can buy a passport, driver's license and vehicle registration from the "Washitaw Nation"--apparently an American Indian nation. Call Rightway Travel at 303-629-9599.

Or, you can buy a nonvalid "camouflage" passport, designed to shield your American nationality from hijackers. These are excellent reproductions of passports from now defunct or renamed nations, such as: British Honduras, Dutch Giana, New Hebrides, Burma, Rhodesia, Ceylon, and Zanzibar. While these will *not* get you into foreign countries, they will probably suffice for intra-U.S.A. documentation. How many cops will know that British Honduras is now Belize? Besides, a *real* British Honduras passport would be valid until it expires-- even if Belize was formed before then.

Don't use your real name. Pick a foreign mail drop as your ID's address. You might even use a disguise for the photos.

A passport (no choice of country), driver's license and two supporting ID's (insurance card, club membership, etc.) sell for Ø399. Write Scope International Ltd., Forestside House, Rowlands Castle, Hants, PO9 6EE, England, UK. I've also seen these passports advertised by other companies.

On *being* a foreigner

Wear foreign clothes--especially shoes. Funky shoes and a Grand Canyon T-shirt says *"tourist"*--which is exactly the idea. Your local youth hostel will have foreign kids passing through. Stop by to learn some foreign color.

Learn the foreign mannerisms. Russians, for example, peel their bananas from the bottom, not top down from the stem. Europeans count 1 to 5 from thumb to pinky. (Only Americans save the thumb for last.) The ✥ hand sign means "✱sshole" in most countries, so foreigners wouldn't use it here to signal "O.K." (When Dan Quayle visited South America as our Vice President, he often flashed an insultingly obscene ✥ to the crowd, to the horror of his hosts.) In a cinema, most foreigners will pass through a row *facing* those already seated, unlike us. Do some research on how "you" are supposed to act.

Know about your foreign country and home town. Know the history, and keep up on current events. If you claim to be from Paris, know who your mayor is, what color the trams are, and what the current nightspots are.

Speak with a *slight* accent--don't overdo it. A *moderate* clumsiness in cadence and syntax is enough. (Most foreigners speak very good English, and you'll be sincerely complimented on yours. Modestly thank them.) The trick to the clothes, accent and mannerisms is to *suggest* foreign status. Let the cop or clerk make the ancillary links himself.

THE FUTURE OF FAKE ID

Rather bleak, actually. Databanks are becoming more sophisticated and better linked. And, hordes of Americans (not to mention illegal aliens) are now using alias ID's to escape bureaucracies and regulations. The feds will soon use this to justify new forms of "unforgeable" ID.

Digital biometric ID

This is real "mark of the beast" stuff, and it's on its way. Such an ID would digitize your body's characteristics (iris, DNA, fingerprint, voiceprint, Human Leukocyte Antigen, etc.). Your number would become "Your Number" on your new ID.

Branding our American soldiers like cattle

The U.S. military already uses such an evil control device called the *Multi-Technology Automated Reader Card*, or MARC. Several soldiers have been court-martialed for refusing to give blood and saliva samples for the DNA registry.

"Your DNA identification number, please?

Other DNA registrants include babies and criminals. Soon, DNA or some other form of biometric ID will be demanded of us all in the guise of either driver's licenses, health cards, worker citizen cards, or the 1994 *"U.S. Card"* which was postponed in 1994 due to public horror.

Project L.U.C.I.D.

Read Ira Levin's *This Perfect Day* to understand what could be in store for us if the Project L.U.C.I.D. goes on-line. Once the human sheep have been branded with the *"Universal Biometrics Card"* (containing 5 *giga*bytes of personal data) they will be tracked by the **Logical Universal Communication Interactive Databank** (L.U.C.I.D.). We are to be tagged like fish, and globally watched like suspected terrorists. *All* of us.

> [L.U.C.I.D. designer] *Dr. Jean-Paul Creusat, M.D., who works on the staff of* Interpol, *a European-based international police agency, and who is also somehow affiliated with the United Nations, involved with two little-known U.S. corporations, Advanced Technology Group and Birkmayer Software, [is] designing a system for a world-wide, criminal justice computer tracking...and control network, to be used by the CIA, FBI, et al.* **All of this he does while claiming to be independent, with funds...being "privately generated."**
> -- Texe Marrs; *Project L.U.C.I.D.,* (1996) p. 36

Please order the above book (ISBN 1-884302-02-5) and *The Mark of the New World Order* by Terry L. Cook (ISBN 0-88368-466-7). You need these two books to understand the times! Today, even *secular* journalists and authors are recognizing the modern parallels to St. John's description of the Beast system.

AT&T's new equipment corporation is called **Lucent** Technologies, which just introduced its new computer operating system **Inferno**, written in language **Limbo** with protocols called **Styx**. (*Three* synonyms for hell is just a *coincidence*...) The *Inferno* network system is designed to make TV's, phones, etc. *interactive* and tied to L.U.C.I.D. **Orwell's *1984* spying telescreen from Hell--I mean *Inferno*.**

My, we're really getting our faces *rubbed* in it, *aren't* we?

Implants for everyone

The basic system consists of an implantable biochip transponder and an external scanning device. The transponders come in various sizes, the smallest of which (at this time--but remember, everything is getting smaller) is about the size of an uncooked grain of rice (11mm). The transponder is a glass tube made of soda lime glass which is known for biocompatibility. During manufacture, this glass tube is hermetically sealed so it is not possible for any body fluids to reach the internal electronics (or vice versa).

There are only three components inside. The first is a computer microchip...which contains the unique ID number which has been etched onto the surface of the microchip. Once the microchip has been encoded, or encrypted, by the manufacturer, it is impossible to alter. The second component is a coil of copper wire wound around a ferrite (iron) core. This coil functions as a tiny radio antenna to pick up the radio signal from the external scanner and to send back the encoded ID number. The third component is a capacitor which...facilitates the signal to and from the microchip.

This type of transponder is a passive device, meaning it has no batteries and never can wear out. It is energized by a low-frequency radio wave from the scanner. Most scanners use a frequency of 125kHz, the signal used in AM medium-wave broadcasting. These low-frequency radio waves can penetrate all solid objects except those made of metal. Electronic ID based on these radio signals is referred to as RFID (Radio Frequency Identification Device). Once the scanner is activated, it digitally displays the decoded ID number on a liquid crystal screen. Destron can encode up to ten digits on their smallest biochip. Texas Instruments has a brand new chip which will allow the encoding of up to nineteen digits. By combining the digits in a variety of combinations, the smallest biochips can be programmed **with up to 34 billion code numbers.** *A spokesman from Trovan says that with the latest technology "the number of possible code combinations is close to one trillion."*

Each transponder comes prepackaged inside a sterilized needle, which is discarded after use. ...In order to prevent the biochip from moving around, one end is sheathed in a polypropylene shell. This coating offers a surface with which fibrous connective tissue begins to bond within 24 hours after injection. **In other words, once the biochip is implanted, it become part of you with an "unlimited lifespan" (Trovan).**

-- Terry L. Cook; *The Mark of the New World Order*, p. 316-7

Whatever the excuse, know that smart cards are merely a temporary expedient in the goal of mass implantation of digital transponder chips. Don't laugh--L.A. County already requires them for all pets. Biochips are now being tested in humans.

Are these implants to be the *"mark of the beast"*?
There's little difference between a MARC *held* in your hand and a mark *implanted* there (Revelation 13:11-18). The really eerie thing about Rev. 13:16 is the **sub**topical, not topical, nature of the mark of the beast: *"And he causeth all, both small and great, rich and poor, free and bond, to receive a mark **in** their right hand, or **in** their foreheads:"*.

The word *"mark"* (*Strong's Exhaustive Concordance of the Bible*, No. 5480) is from the Greek word *charagma* which is connected by *The Expanded Vine's Expository Dictionary of New Testament Words* to **stigma** (*Strong's* No. 4742), in which *Strong's* references *stigma* back to the Greek word **stizo**, which means *"...**to prick, stick, incise, or punch for recognition of ownership**...Scar of service: **a mark**."* Beasts of the beast.

The line in the sand
Future ID's are not really about positive identification. They are really about *control*. Control is a right of *ownership*. Since the Social Security Number was created in 1935, Americans have been herded onto the federal ranch. Those voluntarily branded with an SSN are property of the U.S. government. (Try to *act* like a free person today and you will be judicially thrown back into the cowpen by the scruff of your neck.)

How have we arrived at our putrid state? How have Americans come to be utterly *owned*? How did we accept the haughty demand of government to be licensed for marriage, driving, owning a pet, and conducting a business? **Why didn't we *revolt* when government was still hesitant and timid?**

Now, Europeans call us *"the obedient ones."* (Coming from *them*--the ocean calling the pond "wet"--that's quite an insult.)

Will we take the *"mark"*? Will we be the perfect chattel of the global socialists? If the biometric branding goes forward, then America will obey and suffer without end.

Many Americans simply will *not* tolerate this gross invasion of privacy. I predict that the push for a biometric national ID card will be the final straw for fencesitters. **The national ID card scheme should be *everybody's* line in the sand.** Just say *"NO!"* to Big Brother. Refuse to be branded!

The wimps among our borders should all move to Singapore and get their own mandatory ID card.

FINANCIAL PRIVACY

This will be a big shock to you, but I highly recommend using cash wherever possible. Credit cards and checks, though convenient, create records. Privacy is never convenient.

CREDIT CARDS

Protesting too loudly about [the power of credit card companies] *isn't going to help either, **because the disturbance you kick up is going to end up in one of your files.** And on that come and get it day when you're totally and completely dependent on our card...**you might be left alone without one.***

-- Terry Galanoy, former Director of Communications of VISA International

They're almost a must today, especially to rent cars or reserve hotel rooms. If you already have your VISA or AmExp, don't dump them. Feed them address and phone disinfo. Your credit cards should have little or no activity, and certainly *none* at gun stores, travel agencies, favorite bars and restaurants, or other illuminating places.

If you have no cards, but want some, get them *before* you quit your job and start a cash economy business. Getting cards can be tough, though keeping them is easy if you'll just pay your bills. Perhaps a friend might get a supplement card for you on his account. Avoid the photo credit cards.

Get a foreign credit card

Many foreign banks offer debit VISA's with your "credit" being commensurate with your account balance. Typically, these account cards require an opening balance of at least USØ10,000. Foreign VISA's are great because you're not listed in the domestic databanks, and the records are harder (though not impossible) for the feds to acquire. You can repatriate Ø3-500 per day at ATM's. (ATM's have cameras. Wear a full-face motorcycle helmet with sunglasses during the transaction.)

ecash by DigiCash

Using ecash is like using a virtual ATM. When connecting to it over the Internet, you authenticate ownership of your account and request the amount of ecash you want to withdraw, much like in person. But instead of putting paper cash in your wallet, your software stores the digital cash it obtains on the hard disk of your PC.

[To pay], you confirm the amount, purpose and payee and then your ecash software transfers the [digital] coins from your disk.

*Behind the user interface, your computer actually chooses the serial numbers of the electronic coins based on a random seed. Then it hides them in special encryption envelopes, provides them to the virtual ATM for signing, and removes the envelopes from what is returned--leaving the bank's validating digital signature on the serial numbers. This way, when the bank receives from the shop the coins you spend, it cannot recognize them as coming from any particular withdrawal, because they were hidden in [your encrypted] envelopes during withdrawal. **And thus the bank cannot know when or where you shop or what you buy.***

-- http://www.digicash.com

It's as if anonymous depositors put cash into your account and every "check" has an untraceable payee. The only information your virtual bank account could offer is a history of nameless deposits and withdrawals! While they are many forms of electronic payment, only ecash by DigiCash offers utter privacy.

The Mark Twain bank of St. Louis accepts ecash payments. You could set up an account there, be paid through ecash transactions (just as if some anonymous person deposited cash in your account) and spend ecash, or get ATM paper cash.

CHECKS

*Your canceled checks record the names of your doctors and hospitals, the publications you read, the relatives you help, the religious and charitable activities you support, the volume of business you give your liquor store and the amount you spend on transportation. **The information in canceled checks can be a mirror of your life, a reflection that you do not want seen by the wrong set of eyes.***

-- Robert Ellis Smith; editor of the *Privacy Journal*

I don't use checks. I hate them. First of all, the banks think it's *their* money. Reconciling the account monthly and arguing with Bookkeeping is great fun. Lastly, your privacy goes out the window. Since 1970, banks have been required to microfilm *both* sides of any checks over Ø100. Since sorting those out is too labor-intensive, they simply microfilm them *all* and will turn them over to the government on demand.

While businesses must often use checks, you personally don't have to. Insist on cash, or cash the check at the payor's bank. (Now, many banks are insisting that noncustomers have their *fingerprint* digitally read before cashing a check.) If that bank is far away, endorse it through a friend's account.

Quit using checks! It's the banks' way of creating credit "money" out of nothing. Use cash and M.O.'s--starve them out! Besides, checks bounce and banks are constantly going bust. Use cash for extra safety (as long as the cash is readily accepted, and someday it *won't* be, so be prepared with gold and silver).

ALWAYS BUY THESE WITH CASH

Use cash and concoct a one-time transaction alias if a name if needed. While this list cannot be all-inclusive, it's a good place to start. Think of other items on your own.

● **Guns, ammo and shooting supplies.**
Go to gun shows for anonymous purchases. Have utterly *no* records of gun-related items tied to your name.

● **Books and magazines.**
One's reading list speaks volumes of one's interests, tastes and habits. Be careful of which books you check out at the library. Frequent used bookstores, but don't get chummy. It's preferable to buy gun magazines at the newsstand rather than to subscribe. Isn't privacy worth an extra few dollars a year?

If you don't have an alias with separate address for mail-ordering, then don't order books directly from Loompanics, Eden, etc. in your own name. Go to a local bookstore and prepay your alias order in cash through them. (Know the title, author and ISBN of your book.) When they ask for your phone number, reply that you're just visiting and that you'll call *them*.

● **Travel tickets.**
This is getting harder to do, but I'll cover it later in more detail.

● **Auto parts.**

No use having your make and model of car easily traceable through credit cards or microfilmed checks.

● **Tires and shoes.**

Both leave identifying tracks. You never know what weird situation may arise in which not leaving traceable tracks is advantageous. Since your car's license plate will often be noted on the tire invoice, use an old plate from another car and throw some mud on the expired sticker.

● **Grocery store purchases.**

Their inventories are wonderfully computerized these days. Look at your next receipt and you'll be amazed at the detail recorded. *Exactly* what, where and when is there for checking. Your diet, house cleaning habits and contraceptive usage could be analyzed by sicko government types. (This isn't much of an issue *now*, but the Thought Police is growing. Read *This Perfect Day* by Ira Levin to see where we're probably headed.)

● **Any item which might be returned for a refund.**

If you pay cash, you'll be refunded in cash instead of by check. Keep your receipt.

● **Pets and supplies.**

You don't want vet records of "Whiskers" the cat to be traced to you, so they shouldn't have your address or phone number. Since they'll want an address for the rabies tag, concoct one.

MONEY ORDERS

M.O.'s are lovely. Buy them with cash and no ID is required. They're available practically everywhere. They only cost 25¢ to 99¢. And, for those of you who care, M.O.'s aren't inflationary by adding to the phantom bank credit "money" supply as do checks. M.O.'s are lovely. Use them whenever you must mail payment, or when you don't want to be seen.

Granted, a paper trail *is* created, but records are not sorted by the purchaser's name. The issuer will have the cashed original, the payee's bank will have microfilmed copy, and you might even have the receipt. Unless, however, one knew *where* to start (with the M.O. company, the payee, or your records), there's no picking up the trail. Most often, the payee (who got paid) is the point of investigatory origin.

Mail order houses will record their customers' name and shipping address. If you used an alias and had your UPS package sent to a private mail receiving service--*so what*? The Branch Davidians had *so* much gun stuff UPS'ed right to their door that UPS went to the feds. Use some discretion.

Address-related M.O. payments

If, however, you M.O. paid rent, storage space, utilities or home phone service, then an address *could* be discovered. Even so, how would they know to check your *landlord's* banking records unless they already knew where you lived? (It's easy to catch birds by sprinkling salt on their tails.) These bills can be paid in cash, unless you don't want yourself seen.

For *each* address, buy your M.O.'s from the *same* place to avoid comingling information (domicile with storage unit, for example). Never buy consecutive M.O.'s from any one store, and don't use the same store more than once every six months.

What about the receipts?

Keep them *only* if you might need to later prove payment. Address-oriented receipts (i.e., utilities, rent, home phone, etc.) should be kept *at that address* and not in your car or on your person. When you buy an addressed-oriented M.O., put the receipt in a locked briefcase as soon as you get to your car. **Don't leave them in your wallet or purse.** You might get arrested for some old traffic ticket and your address get discovered. Once home, transfer the receipt inside. Be thorough and stay sharp.

Receipts for sensitive mail order products should not be kept at home, in your car or on your person. I have a separate location away from home to store soon-to-be-burned receipts.

Yeah, I know, all this is a *pain*. Well, privacy *is* a pain. If you're not up to it, then just go get a checking account. Fishbowl *"Yes, Sir!"* living is *easy*--that's why so many people don't *mind* it. But hey, only *learning* to live privately is difficult. Once learned, it's merely tedious and somewhat inconvenient.

Watch out for "structuring"

Since any cash transaction exceeding Ø3,000 in a single day is reportable on a *Currency Transaction Report* (CTR), people simply spread out large purchases over several days or purchase orders. It is a crime (called "structuring") to intentionally avoid the reporting requirement. **Structuring** makes it a crime to *avoid* a crime. Structuring works like this: let's say a "Peeping Tom" law was passed which prohibited looking in somebody's window for more than 10 consecutive seconds per minute. Anyone who innocently looked in a window for 6 seconds one minute, and 5 seconds another could be charged with "structuring" by splitting up 11 seconds of looking into more than one minute--thus circumventing the "Peeping Tom" statute. Crazy, isn't it? I am *not* advocating that you engage in "structuring." I'm merely pointing out that it *is* done frequently. Your call.

LOANS & MORTGAGES

Try to avoid them. Investment capital is one thing, but to pay interest on *depreciating* goods is a financial sin. Worse still is all the information you'll have to divulge on the application. Save up and buy it outright. *Earn* more money--don't borrow it.

IRAs, 401Ks & KEOGHs

These tax-deferred savings plans are congressionally created corrals to lure in private pensions. One day soon, Congress will mandate that a portion (ever to increase, of course) must be "invested" in Treasury securities--for your "protection," you see.

Therefore, you should plan to drop out at some point, even if it means taking the 10% early withdrawal penalty. Until then, you can *truly* invest your capital in gold coins which are stored for you by a trustee. While the IRS won't let you keep them yourself, it beats having your life's savings left at risk in the stock market.

GOLD & SILVER COINS

This is *real* money with perfect intrinsic value. Everything else merely *hopes* to be accepted by sellers. Buy *bullion* coins because when gold and silver coins are again outlawed, few will pay any numismatic premium for your contraband $20 St. Gaudens, and no hick will have *heard* of PCGS. (And even if he *had*, he'll bicker over grading, *"Looks lahk MS62 tuh me!"*) Buy with cash at gun and coin shows. Split up your hoard. (See chapter 11 of my *Boston on Surviving Y2K* for a full discussion on gold and silver coins, numismatic and bullion.)

PRIVACY & TAXES

The chief purpose of the [income] *tax is not financial,* **but social.** *It is not primarily to raise money for the State,* **but to regulate the [U.S.]** *citizen.*
   -- Rep. Samuel McCall (R-MA), on the 16th Amendment

My first book, *Good-Bye April 15th!*, was published in 1992. A lot has happened since then. The untax procedure I outlined is very aggressive and public. While I've heard of nothing to dispute the legal technique involved, untaxation is apparently no longer enjoying all of its earlier success.

In retrospect, I wish that I had written *Bulletproof Privacy* before *Good-Bye April 15th!* It is preferable to first change domiciles and shield your assets *before* attempting to untax yourself. I assumed this would be obvious so I did not stress the point. Unfortunately, overconfidence in the government's evidently checkmated legal position regarding its limited tax jurisdiction caused some people to act too boldly. What they didn't take into account is that the IRS would simply ignore or disallow the untax paperwork and proceed to seize assets. While no reader of mine has written me with such horror story, I've heard of this happening to followers of *other* untax authors. (I won't name names because I don't want to leave anybody *out.*)

I'm moving into areas which I consider to be more practical and workable. Roadside rights, privacy, the future and effectiveness of the Constitution, and parallel financial systems which offer anonymity. And, quite frankly, I've grown tired of untaxation and jurisdiction and sovereignty. They are tedious, draining subjects to research, and I won't compete with the current chorus of untax, me-too "Patrioteers."

    If the government insists that you *are* subject to its tax jurisdiction--what *legal* recourse do you have? The courts are staffed by government employees. On whose side do you imagine they will rule? The government *knows* that we've finally cracked their statute fraud wide open, and they're not about to say, *"O.K., yuh got us!"* (Somebody show me a victory check from a Title 42 suit.) We cannot force the government to accept legal responsibility, much less punishment, for its fraud.

    Untaxation worked within its opportunity window when there were enough people involved for a "critical mass" of quality procedure, but not *too* many to panic the government. *The government is now panicking.* Informationally speaking, the dam has cracked. While unfixable, the feds *can* build levees to prevent the water of truth from spilling over the bank of mass ignorance. Frantic sandbagging will be the feds post-1996 response to untaxation. They will *de facto* circumvent our *de jure* chipping away at the statutory dam. Mark my words: the flood of legal proaction *will* be contained. We hadn't *enough* chisels.

    I was admittedly too optimistic and idealistic to clearly foresee this. We *all* were. **Now, let's get *realistic.*** Dracula is wearing sunglasses to the blinding sun of truth. We're not going to win this just because we know the difference between *"citizen"* and "Citizen." Understanding the Buck Act of 1940 won't bring the lawless feds to their knees. This war is now beyond law and the courts--the judges say so.

    Quality Patriot briefs and motions are being dismissed out of hand as irrelevant or inflammatory. *Pro per* defendants are being sent away for psychiatric observations, and *kept* there. The government has learned that we've done little effective *so far* to halt its tyranny. When the FBI can shoot nursing mothers in the face and burn children alive in their homestead church--*without punishment*--just how scared do you think the IRS is of your *paperwork?* Wake up! Clinton just got *reelected!* Tyranny is on a *roll.* We've lost the untax round.

    So, burrow down and plan for a rainy decade or two. Let's not get wiped out in a fruitless legal battle where we've committed even our reserves. Legal forays are one thing; kamikaze attacks are another. Let's wise up. The feds will not back down just because we can write a 27 CFR or 4 USC *"Simon says."* They are too deeply committed to give up *that* easily, and it's time we faced up to it. This *won't* be a quick or easy victory.

YOUR MAIL

RECEIVING YOUR MAIL

How you set up your mail is as important as your phone. The primary rules are: ❶ Have your senders omit their return address and use yours instead, and ❷, *never* receive mail at your house. *Ever!* To receive mail there first requires that you give out your house address (or "mailing location", for you legal types)--something you never want to do. Well, then, what are the alternatives to getting mail at the end of your driveway?

How to create a red herring address

Sometimes a P.O. box will *not* be accepted--they (DMV, P.O., library, credit cards, cell phone provider, etc.) want a *street* address. You want to provide a *prima facie* legitimate address which doesn't lead anywhere. Don't be a smartass and say *"1060 W. Addison"* in Chicago, which is Wrigley Field. You want to cost the investigator precious time. A good red herring is something that *can't* be discounted with a simple phone call.

The country road ploy

Here's an original Boston tip. Use some fictitious box number on a very remote rural route, preferably way down some dirt road. Pick an RR which is *really* far flung (see the map in your phone book). Buy a mailbox, affix some decals for your number and nail it to a 4x4 post when you are certain the mail carrier won't drive by. Wipe off all fingerprints. Don't use it for a mail drop, and never return. Most rural route mail carriers are contracted help and not actual U.S.P.S. employees (quasi-feds). They'll most likely stuff your phony mailbox without asking why it just appeared on their route.

This address *looks* bonafide, yet *really* wastes an investigator's time because it *is* "bonafide." An RR box number is time-consuming to check out, much less *stake* out. Imagine all the fun he'll have living in his car, waiting for you to pick up your mail. Have some junk mail sent there, and some postcards from Gunter in Vienna asking when you're coming over. Every minute spent on false leads means a minute lost on real leads.

"Which number, please?"

If the RR box is too much trouble, almost as good is the address of a large apartment complex (omitting any room number). Check the Yellow Pages or a collective brochure on the city's apartments. This address can't be easily discounted as false, even by interviewing the manager and the tenants.

Good, old General Delivery (G.D.)

This is a free service. Smaller post offices provide quicker and more personal attention than big city stations. Your mail will be returned to the sender after 30 days, so be diligent about picking it up. Usually, some form of ID will be required, though not always (especially if you're a known regular). If you make a several month habit of general delivery, some clerks will try to make you get a P.O. box. Though I haven't researched the Domestic Mail Manual (D.M.M.) for any time limits on G.D., you might check it out.

The main disadvantage to G.D. is that you can only pick up your mail in person during lobby hours. This is inconvenient and demands excessive transactional exposure. Therefore, use G.D. for infrequent tasks, and vary the P.O.'s.

If you're overseas, you can receive mail c/o any American Express office. If you've an AmEx card or traveler's checks, the service is free--otherwise it's a buck or two. Get the AmEx listing of all their offices and let your people know where you'll be and when. I've used this service often, and it's a great way to keep your foreign address private. AmEx is also quite helpful with other traveling needs (language barriers, directions, etc.). They'll also cash a cardmember's U.S.A. check! Such takes at least two weeks to clear, giving you that much more locational privacy over the real-time ATM's.

The P.O. box

I like small town P.O. boxes. They're fairly private and dirt cheap. The yearly box fee is as little as Ø8. Outside large cities, a P.O. will leave the front door open so you can pick up your mail after hours. Choose a P.O. which has after hours lock boxes for oversized parcels (the greatest postal innovation in years, besides self-adhesive stamps). Since there's no national registry, you could have many boxes across the country.

The application procedure is no big worry. Minimal ID is required and a local address. Do *not* conjure up an address, because it'll likely be noticed as such. Use my RR box or apartment complex ploy.

Helpful previous boxholders

You will undoubtedly receive a bit of mail for previous boxholders. Remember their names. Why not receive a thing or two in *their* name? Even though it arrived in *your* box, you can easily disavow it as a stranger's mail. Don't get them into trouble, but don't pass up this free and convenient alias.

The private mailbox

These are commercially operated alternatives to the U.S.P.S. The yearly box fees start at Ø80--at least twice than a comparable P.O. box. For this extra expense, you get to call in and check for mail, plus have the convenience of a fax number and UPS shipping/receiving. Since you *never* want UPS packages delivered to your house, having them sent to a private receiver is a great service (though you don't have to be a boxholder and can simply pay Ø1-3 per package instead).

Even though postal form 1583 (*Application for Delivery of Mail through Agent*) doesn't require an ID, these companies are more stringent about ID than the P.O. Some even photocopy the applicant's ID, or expressly warn that no warrant shall be deemed necessary for cops to obtain information. (Mail Boxes Etc. is notorious for this.) Visit your available services and choose wisely. If run by elderly people or immigrants, *beware*--they'll typically bend over for any badge that walks in the door. Find an independent *nonchain* store. The best staff are funky-type college kids. They dislike authority and will rarely give out private info to the law (unless strongly threatened or well-paid for it). *Right on!*

The mail forwarding services

Most private mailbox services also forward mail, and not just for their boxholders. Some companies are purely forwarders. For postage and Ø1 fee per piece, they'll send on your mail. Simply address and stamp your letter and nest it inside a larger envelope with a Ø1 bill. No fuss, no muss.

To *receive* mail from a forwarder, you must obviously give them some address. You can forward through other forwarders, but don't use too many (over 3) or else your mail takes much longer, is at more risk to loss or theft, and looks like hell when it finally arrives. You can even mail forward through dozens of foreign countries: Costa Rica, Germany, England, etc. Get a copy of Budd's Remailing List from Eden Press.

A word or two of caution

Some basic rules: Pick up your mail at infrequent and varied times. Never sign for certified or registered mail unless you expect it. Any mail not for you, throw it away--don't remail it. If you've reason to believe that your P.O. is being watched, have your mail forwarded, or picked up by a friend, or let it sit for a while until they give up and quit the stakeout.

If you're ever *really* sought after, and they can't find you, they have some clever tricks. Assuming you've rented a box and they've staked out the application's bogus RR box or apartment address to no avail, the only alternative is to try and catch you at the mail drop itself.

There are two general methods. The first is to have a clerk tip them off the next time you visit the lobby. If this happens, the chances are good that you'll notice the clerk's change in attitude towards you. They're clerks, not actors. If he has to *"check something in back"* and leaves his window, *get out.*

If the clerk route is not deemed reliable (or isn't possible because a private investigator has no official capacity to arrange it), then they'll have to hang out across the street and wait for you. If you never check your mail more than once a week at varied times, the stakeout will be a *real* drag.

If your description is vague or unknown, they'll send a distinctive package to you which must be picked up at the window (i.e., a long, yellow mailing tube which won't even fit in the parcel lockboxes). If you ever receive such a surprise, *don't take it outside*--somebody is probably waiting for you to generously ID yourself. You should refuse it, which is sound policy with unexpected parcels from unknown people.

The self-addressed, stamped envelope (SASE)

Frequently, readers will send me letters asking for my reply and helpfully enclose a SASE. (I answer these first.) While I happily use their SASE, I *never* lick the envelope. I use a foam moistener instead. Although I trust my readers, some nasty character could spike the glue with some unpleasantness and I wouldn't know it until it was too late. Such caution is not paranoia, but simply studied prudence.

Be alert to unusual patterns or delays in receiving mail.

In a "mail cover" operation, officials will photocopy your received envelopes for return addresses and meter ID's. In the 1960's, the feds caught many people with undeclared foreign bank accounts simply by tracing the metered mail to Swiss banks. No mail on Saturday and a big batch on Monday can signal a mail cover, as nonpostal feds don't work on Saturdays.

SENDING YOUR MAIL

How you send your mail is also important. Speed of service and the postmark are sometimes vital criteria.

How to send from "A" and get a "B" postmark

You can have somebody (friend or company) forward it on as described above. Or, in some areas a big city P.O. will send a truck out to pick up rural *outside* dropboxes. Although I live an hour away from Austin, I use a box which is serviced by an Austin P.O. truck. The way to check this for sure is to buy some prestamped, blank postcards from any P.O. and send them to yourself, having notated each card with which dropbox it was sent from. Remember, this distant postmarking is only for *outside* dropboxes, not those inside a P.O.

Low exposure mailing

Sensitive letters or cash should be wrapped in foil, as certain sprays (e.g., Freon) will make the envelope temporarily opaque. Tape all flaps and sides with your initial or code underneath (so the receiver will know *you* taped it). Don't get funky on how you address your mail. Sovereign style addresses are of marginal legal value (at best), and will only draw attention to the letter. Use block letters in black pen on plain envelopes. Use the *recipient's* address (if you're *sure* of it) as the "return" address. Some people have a P.O. *and* a street address. Use one as the sendee and the other as the sender--that way, even if you forget to affix postage, they'll still get it.

I prefer stamping my own mail to avoid visiting a clerk's window. You'll need a rate sheet, a scale and many assorted stamps. Avoid using postage meters unless absolutely necessary. Each meter has an ID number, tied to the renter.

Also, I think it's wise to send mail from a P.O. other than where you receive. If this isn't convenient, then send your mail from a dropbox. (Be sure to note the pickup times so that you don't needlessly cost your mail an extra day.) I'd never drop off mail at a private mailbox company. Use U.S.P.S. boxes only.

Outgoing mail requiring postal clerk attention should be carefully thought through. Plan ahead where that return receipt should arrive, what the contents are, etc. Sometimes you can't avoid having to visit a clerk. Most are very nice, however, some are quite nosey. If you don't want them to in-spect your mail after you've stepped away, simply ask for appropriate *stamp* postage (as opposed to metered, which cannot be handed back to you). Since this is a little uncommon, use the excuse that the piece isn't *quite* ready to go yet as you have to first verify the address, *blah, blah, blah*. Walk out with it and send from a dropbox.

PRIVACY & THE PHONE

It is my view that, besides your own tongue, the telephone is the instrument most potentially compromising of your privacy. More investigations have begun (and succeeded) with information derived from numbers called and conversations conducted. If you will learn to govern how, when and to whom your calls are made, the difficult task of privacy will then largely be accomplished. For Americans, however, this is an exceedingly inconvenient habit to perform over many years.

When telephones were newly invented, a budding futurist was laughed at because he envisioned the day when every *town* would have one. Today, multiple phone lines per *household* is quite common, hence the clunky new area codes.

The proliferation of cellular phones is only the latest wave in personalized telecommunication. Within 10 years, they will have gone the way of the 8-track tape when Motorola's Iridium system (or something like it) finally becomes operational. Named "Iridium" after its atomic number of 77, the plan is to have 7 orbits containing 11 satellites each. Good-bye "long-distance" calls. Instead, calls to your Iridium number will be linked by satellite and therefore "distance independent." The downside to this is, no matter where you are on the *planet,* your location will be always known while your Iridium phone is on.

Frankly, it's just not *practical* to be without telephones. Besides, to be without one seems odd and suspicious. So, it's vital to have a phone number for expediency's sake and not to draw attention to yourself. This can be accomplished with little sacrifice in privacy, as I'll explain shortly.

METHODS OF COMPROMISE

I'll list them in increasing order of severity.

Your listed phone number

Gee, now the whole *world* knows where you live and how to call you at anytime. Sadly, a nonpublished number is no stumbling block for the resourceful, though it will hamper the random public. In truth, it's merely a marketing scam to pilfer an extra Ø3 a month from single women.

Your phone records

Long-distance records are easily obtainable by officials and private investigators. Also, and not widely known, your *local* calling records (Message Unit Details, or MUD's) are kept for at least 6 months *and will be analyzed* during any serious investigation. *Many* criminals have been convicted because of their MUD's.

To my knowledge, the records of your *incoming* calls are not routinely kept. Such requires the following device.

The "pen register" to learn of your network

This is like a mail-cover for telephones. It notates the time, date, number dialed and duration of your outgoing calls. More sophisticated units work with Caller ID and notate your *incoming* calls as well. Pen registers are often, though not always, operated directly from the phone company. The feds, however, enjoy dedicated lines to their buildings.

The "tap" to record the conversation

In the analog days, placing a tap (or, "trap") on a line required the assistance of AT&T. Today, digital switching centers and touch-tone phones are in use for at least 95% of the American system. This modernization has brought benefits to the public, as well as to government snoops.

The feds can activate a tap on a line simply by calling a central number and then entering the number to be tapped. Even still, taps are fairly uncommon as they are quite labor intensive. *Somebody* has to listen in, though the feds have computers with voice recognition which print out the conversations.

The "trace"

In the days of mechanical switching and rotary dial phones it required 30-90 seconds to complete a trace, but not any more. With digital equipment, a trace is *instantaneous*. (Caller ID is merely a commercially available trace.) Whenever you call 800 #'s, 911, the police, the operator, or high-level officials, your number is immediately displayed--unless you're "phreaking" the system (as in the movie *Ransom*).

PRIVACY MEASURES

You *must* get 2 voice mail (VM) numbers

No real privacy is possible without voice mail numbers--trust me on this. VM#1 is your "official" or "public" number instead of a home phone. Remember, this number is your *public* number, so *think through any possible linkage* to your private life, address and number. VM#2 (with pager notification) is for good friends only. Establish it under an alias, or have a friend sign up instead. If alias established, have the bills go somewhere *other* than to addresses under your own name.

The service will cost Ø10-15 per month, depending on where you live and the features you want. I would opt for the full package which has longer message length and retention, and pager notification (when a caller leaves a message, your pager is beeped and you know within a seconds to check in).

To the caller, it sounds like an answering service. Messages are moderately safe behind a security code (usually 4 digits) of your choosing. Do not use obvious permutations of your voice mail number, your SSN, birthday, etc. Change the code often, especially during times of heightened alert. If things are *really* edgy, turn off the pager notification to keep its number private and communicate by code (see 12/5-8).

Keep your greeting short and simple without leaving your name: *"Hello. Sorry we're not here right now. Please leave a short message after the beep. Thank you."* **For ultra-privacy,** have a friend record the VM#2 greeting *for* you so your voice isn't connected with the number. Instruct your callers not to babble sensitive information (or unnecessarily leave their name and number if you know them by voice).

From any touch-tone phone you can check your messages, or change your greeting, security code and even the number to be notified when you've received a message. Once you've picked up a message, erase it immediately! Even though the system can save messages for days, save them yourself in your password-protected PDA. **For ultra-privacy,** do not call in from your home phone--always use distant and varied pay phones. You don't want an unknown pen register to notate incoming calls from sensitive numbers.

If you're using aliases, be certain that each personality has its *own* voice mail number and billing address. Watch out for any crossovers. Compartmentalization is the key.

You must also get a pager

To eliminate going to a separate pager company and its additional exposure, get your pager from the VM#2 folks. (Your "public" VM#1 should *not* have pager notification. Keep VM#1 a complete dead-end.) Since pagers are so versatile, private and vital, I discuss them in Chapter 12, *Privacy With Pagers.*

Why not skip the voice mail and use *only* a pager?

I've tried it. First of all, Grandma won't learn how to use your pager, anyway. Neither will half your family and a third of your friends. Pagers are about as personal as smoke signals and classified ads. And, it's difficult to leave a good-natured dirty message on a pager, so they're no fun, either.

Secondly, it *looks suspicious.* It's counterproductive to let your privacy measures draw attention to yourself. The only people who seem to have *only* a pager are drug dealers, and that's the *last* group you want to appear associated with.

You want to have a normal looking phone number and street address. As long as this *veneer* of normality is kept, few people and companies will ever think to inquire further.

How private are cellular phones?

When powered up and waiting on standby, cell phones emit a *"Here I am!"* signal so that the system will send calls through the nearest cellular transmitter. This signal can be DF'ed (directional finding) to within at least a city block. Since not all areas have the capabilities to do that, a law was passed to require such by 1998. (This is ostensibly to locate incapacitated 911 callers--hah! Big Brother is truly a *caring* sort of guy.)

A sneaky scheme which might work for you.

One of my readers came up with something clever. Since he lives way out in the country with no phone, miles from the nearest pay phone, he got a cell phone with voice mail and pager notification. He leaves his cell phone off and waits for the pager to notify him of a new message. He then powers up the cell phone and accesses his voice mail with no airtime charge. Some calls he returns by cell phone, others he returns later from a pay phone. The Ø35 per month for service, he says, is a bargain compared to driving back and forth to pick up his messages-- most of which do not warrant a special trip into town. Special friends page him first with a preassigned code that tells him to turn on his phone immediately for their incoming call.

This all strikes me as pretty ingenious, though cellular numbers have a unique exchange (i.e., 555-....) which may be too indiscreet for some folks to use as their only voice mail.

Also, I reminded him that all cellular transmissions are easily overheard with scanners. If a target's call is more than a minute or two, one can find his channel amongst dozens of others. Even though the 800 MHz cellular frequencies have been locked out of post-1994 scanners, it's usually a simple matter to clip a lead or remove a chip to restore reception (the older Radio Shack PRO-43's are supremely easy to modify). So, keep your cellular discussions discreet, because...

At least Cellular One digitally records *all* calls.

They do this (ostensibly) so that you cannot disavow call charges, whether incoming or outgoing. After 30-90 days, how-ever, when past bills are considered correct and unassailable the phone company should have no *evidential* reason to retain the recordings--but do you think they *erase* them? *Nooooo...*

Calling records

Detailed records are kept of outgoing calls (like visible MUD's), but no overt records are kept on the phone number of incoming calls. **If you have a cell phone, use *great* caution and discipline in whom you call.** Using a prepaid calling card (more on this in a bit) will only show its 800 number and not the number you call *through* their system. If you're far away from a pay phone and *must* use your cellular to call a sensitive number, you could message his pager (assuming he had one) or arrange a ring-twice-hang-up code for him to call you back. As long as he doesn't answer, your outgoing call won't show up on your records, and his incoming won't either (except generically as *"Incoming Call"*).

Lock your cell phone

First, change the 3 digit lock/unlock code and the 6 digit security code (required for programming functions) and either remember those codes or store them in an encrypted file. Then, program your phone to power up always in the locked mode--requiring the 3 digit unlock code before use.

Cell phones and notebook computers

For *ultra*-privacy, use a laptop computer with cellular modem, PGPfone (**http://web.mit.edu/network/pgpfone/**) or Nautilus. Even if the NSA *could* crack a 1,024 bit RSA key (which I highly doubt), it would take months or years. Your phone conversation probably isn't *that* important.

> [Nautilus] *uses a computer's audio hardware to digitize and play back your speech, using its own built-in speech compression functions. It encrypts the compressed speech, using your choice of the Blowfish, Triple DES, or IDEA block ciphers, and transmits the encrypted packets over your modem to the receiving computer. At the receiving end, the process reverses.* [It's] *half-duplex, so it requires a key stroke to switch between talking and listening.*
> -- Janet Endrijonas; *Data Security,* pp. 158-9

Minimum hardware for Nautilus: 386DX25 PC's with a Soundblaster-compatible sound card (PC sound cards won't work as Nautilus uses the ISA bus) and 9600 bps modem. Celluar calls work better at 4800bps using a fast CPU (486DX2-66 or better). Email them at **nautilus@lila.com** or get it free at:

> **ftp://ftp.csn.org/mpj/README**, or
> **ftp://ripem.msu.edu/pub/crypt/GETTING ACCESS**

Using a cellular sacrifices *numeric* privacy as called numbers appear on your bill (and possibly locational, if you're being DF'ed). Using a landline sacrifices *locational* privacy, but at least the callee's number won't appear on *your* records. For a landline, you'll have plug into somebody's phone jack, since acoustical modems are not fast enough for PGPfone. (Kinkos, hotels, etc. often have phone jacks at private workdesks.)

An acoustical modem of 4800bps *could* be used with a 486DX2-66 (or better) powered Nautilus. With this rig, you could make encrypted calls to and from *pay phones.* Heh!

For secure telephonic data transmission, there's the encryption fax/modem **SafeDial V.34** PC card from RACAL (800-
RACAL-55).   Callees will also need this card--sort of like the
Enigma machine.   Or, you could use a normal fax/modem and
send data encrypted by hardware PC card.   While they're Ø225-
550, these cards are amazing:

CyrptCard from Techmatics	(703-802-8300)
iPower card from NatSemi	(408-721-6601)
Session Key from SCI	(416-798-9600)
SmartDisk from SmartDisk	(941-263-3475)
CryptaPlus Card from Telequip	(603-598-1300)
LYNKS Privacy Card from Spyrus	(800-542-6522)

If these cards seem the answer, do your research and spend
whatever the best card costs.   Warning: anybody going to all
this trouble, however, had better be ready for some eventually
very serious investigation and surveillance.

What about the Clipper chip?

This is the feds' belated response to private encryption
technology.   The silicon Clipper (or Capstone) chip would go in
every new phone, fax machine, modem, etc. It houses the classified (rather than public) algorithm Skipjack which creates a law
enforcement access field (LEAF) to selected (translation: government) escrow agencies.   Meaning, the DoJ can tell an escrow
agency to release the key to your phone's built-in hardware encryption.   Release it to whom?   Any law enforcement agency
which satisfies a mere "need to know" (forget about the 4th
Amendment).   Basically, Clipper conversations are secure *until*
the government takes an interest in them.

Am I worried? Nah! The cat's already out of the bag. Encryption software is prevalent on the Net. If you used an unap-
proved, private encryption envelope, then it'll probably be
flagged--but if you enclose it *within* the Clipper envelope, they'll
never know it unless they open it. Even if we were forced to use
Clipper, simply take phone conversation A, encrypt it privately
to B, and encrypt B with Clipper to C--using Clipper as a mere
envelope around an envelope. The feds break into their own envelope expecting to read the letter--but all they get is an un-
openable internal envelope!   Real time surveillance is
impossible, and that's exactly the idea. *Tee, hee.*

Your listing--if you *must* have a home phone

If you must list your number, at least have your address omitted. Or, the phone company can list your number in another *name*--they don't care as long as they've got a viable billing name and address. I would list it in another name rather than getting a nonpublished listing in your own name, for two reasons: it's *free*, and a call to directory assistance won't have your real name in their records (thus, the caller won't learn that ❶ you're in such-and-such area, and ❷ you have a phone).

For ultra-privacy, have a friend establish the service in his name. Understandably, he may want a cash deposit up front. It's not so unusual for "A" to be on the rental agreement, and "B" to have the phone--especially in college towns.

If nobody is willing to establish service for you, use an alias. Though increasingly difficult, it's still possible. You'll have to pay a several hundred dollar deposit and explain why you don't have a social security number (i.e., you're just starting college and have never had a job, you're from overseas, etc.). Know beforehand that any new number so suspiciously established will be secretly listened in on by the phone company for several weeks. Keep it cool.

Regardless of how or by whom the service was established, you must always realize that those ten digits are physical locators for your house. **Once the number has been linked to you, you can be visited at *any* time.**

Therefore, think long and hard before you get a home phone. If the combination of voice mails, pager and cell phone absolutely will not work for you, then at least get VM#1. Do *not* print your home number on checks, business cards, etc. Do *not* give it out to strangers, prospective dates, classified ad listings, shops, credit card companies, public officials, distant relatives, etc. The only people who should have it are *extremely* close friends and family members, *and even then* do not entrust it to them unless you really must (for emergency purposes, etc.). They should call you from pay phones to avoid making MUD's.

Still, I can't stress this enough: **if you're into low-key living and invisible domiciles--*don't get a home phone*.** Give the cell phone/voice mail/pager combination a fair, *first* try. Cell phones are now *free* with a 12 month contract, and you'll get at least 90 free monthly minutes for the Ø35 deal.

Your calling records

Since anybody who *really* wants your records can get them, the only thing you can do is not *create* them. While this might seem to defeat the purpose of having a phone, such isn't too inconvenient with a bit of forethought and discipline.

Local calls

There are certain local numbers you should *never* call from home: your own voice mails, travel agencies, gun stores, doctors' offices, banks, credit card companies, and "sensitive" friends. Imagine which people and companies you don't want to be connected with by *your* MUD's, or through *their* Caller ID. Damark sells a **Caller ID Blocker** for Ø19.99 (800-729-9000; stock #428874), though *"not available"* in West Virginia, Tennessee, Mississippi, Louisiana or California.

Toll-free 800 and 888 calls

Just because they don't show up on your long-distance records doesn't mean that no records exist. For recordkeeping purposes, these are retained as MUD's. Also, a word of caution: most companies with toll-free numbers also have ANI (Automatic Number Identification), a sort of Caller ID. If you call them from your home they'll make an internal record of where you live. To be safe, use a pay phone for *all* toll-free calls.

Long-distance calls

Since it looks suspicious to have utterly *no* long-distance calls on your bill, make a couple of harmless, generic ones each month. **For ultra-privacy,** never call family and friends.

Use prepaid long-distance calling cards!

These are the greatest privacy innovation in years. Long popular in Europe, they've finally hit our shores. For Ø5-100 you can buy long-distance credit on a disposable card. The higher the denomination, the lower the rate (from 33-20¢ per minute). Calling 50 miles or 5,000 miles away costs the same. (The cheapest rate I've so far seen is 20¢ per minute.)

Although different grocery and drug stores sell their own versions, they all work the same way. To place a call, dial the company's master 800 number, then the card's unique number, and then the number you're calling. You'll be told how much credit the card has left and how many minutes remain. Depending on the company, it takes 35-50 seconds to connect your number. (Try several companies as the quality of service varies.) Usually, you'll get a *"One minute remaining!"* warning before being cut off.

Once used up, *burn* **the card. Do not "throw it away" and** *never* **recharge it with your credit card.** (This was one of Timothy McVeigh's many tactical mistakes.) I recommend burning the card immediately after entering the number into your password-protected PDA or encrypted notebook.

Since even 20¢ per minute adds up, you should generally use the card to make the connection and have your party call you back (unless you cannot trust him with your location, or you don't want the call on *his* long-distance records). Many pay phones still display their number and allow incoming calls, but test them first by calling them yourself or asking the operator to try ringing you back if the pay phone is a singleton.

How *private* are these services?

Good question. It would be an easy feat for the card company to use ANI and link where you're calling *from* with where you're calling to. However, if you make a perfect habit of using only pay phones (and varied ones at that), then such will offer nothing but your general location.

I heard a story about the mother of a runaway girl who asked an FBI friend to trace the home phone to learn where the girl was calling from. Even though the girl was using prepaid cards, the feds *allegedly* traced her calls within hours to pinpoint her location. While I'm not totally discounting their capability to do exactly this, for several reasons I am skeptical about this *particular* story. I discuss it only because it *could* be true. Who knows, the feds themselves could be operating one massive calling-card company under the guise of a dozen commercial names. The sudden proliferation of these calling-cards since 1993 *is* somewhat suspicious. *Cuidado.*

What you *could* do is daisy chain your extremely sensitive calls through two or more of these services. Dial up service A, through A dial up service B, and from B dial your number. Tracing back from your callee will get B's number. Tracing back from B *might,* or might *not,* effectively get A's number--much less your pay phone number. It will at least muddy the trail.

Whether or not companies keep a record of a card's called numbers, I can't say for sure. I would suspect that they do, at least for a few months. **For ultra-privacy,** use separate cards for *each* frequently called sensitive number. Use different companies for each alias. Some calls are business and some are personal--each kind should have their *own* card from *different* companies. Such measures are extreme, but you'll get what you pay for. Half-assed measures will give you half-assed privacy.

One final thought: I wouldn't bet the store on these cards. They are at *least* a buffer to routine, low-level snooping--but that may be *all* they can do. The feds and the phone companies are quite powerful and sophisticated, and if they get together against you, all bets are off. Be very careful about whom you call from the same card, and from the same pay phone. **If you create *possible* links, the links *will* be made if the heat is *really* on. *Count* on it.** Think things through, draw it out, be thorough and consistent. Your freedom depends on it.

The wise use of pay phones

Just because it's a pay phone doesn't mean you can blab with complete abandon. First, consider the *brand* of pay phone. I would trust personally an off-brand over a Bell phone.

Then, there's *location*. Some suspect pay phone locations are: jails, airports and close proximity, bus and train stations, hotels, casinos, nightclubs with a notoriously criminal clientele, government buildings (including post offices), and any quasi-official institution.

If the brand and location do not ring any warning bells, be sure that it can receive incoming calls and that you can speak in privacy with being overheard. Find *at least* a dozen more like pay phones and alternate their usage. **Never use the *same* phone for different calling-cards or personalities.**

For ultra-privacy, never use a pay phone nearby your home, office, hotel, etc. This is an obvious hassle, but I'll be the first to tell you: **privacy *ain't* convenient!** For instance, *if they know the pay phone*, they'll scour that area's hotels, motels, restaurants, etc. *If they know your general location*, they'll get the records of all nearby pay phones and tap the ones they think you use regularly.

This is a common investigation procedure which has yielded much fruit. In *The Silent Brotherhood*, members of the "Order" bought cheap used cars for their getaway vehicles and dumped them. After an armored car robbery, the feds found one of the getaway cars and interviewed the prior owner. He recalled that the buyer asked directions from such-and-such motel. The feds then got the MUD's from every pay phone in that motel's area and found which one the car seller had been called *from*. Analyzing the rest of that phone's records, the FBI learned where the Order's out-of-state headquarters were. It all took a while, but time is *usually* on the side of the investigator.

The Order's mistakes were: *buying* their getaway cars and thus showing their face, calling the sellers from a nearby pay phone, asking for directions from their own motel, and using the same pay phone to call home. Loose ends always provide triggers, and enough triggers will crack *any* case.

Don't get *lazy*. Make your call just before you *leave* the area, not when you arrive. Don't use any nearby trashcans. *Never* use a pay phone at any frequented location where you are known or recognized (i.e., bar, laundromat, car wash, store, etc.), or at locations which have security cameras (i.e., gov't buildings, banks, liquor stores, etc.). Consider using one phone card per callee, and never using a pay phone more than once, or for successive calls. Call your party (preferably at his pager) from one pay phone with coins, and have him call *you* at another pay phone in another town. Yeah, I *know* it's inconvenient, but that's the deal. **Don't get lazy. Make *every* pay phone call a dead-end street which leads *nowhere*.** Nobody *saw* you there, nobody *knows* you there, no successive calls were made, you left nothing at the scene, you *left* immediately after hanging up and wiping off prints--and you'll never *return* there.

The wise use of all other phones

When using a home phone with a redial button, dial that phone's own number as your last call and hang up. This prevents somebody from redialing your last party. Avoid cordless phones--they are overheard without warrant by scanners.

If any phone is within 100 feet of a sensitive conversation, unplug the handset (not the phone itself). Although the phone will still ring, this disconnects the mike and thwarts the "infinity" technique by covert types in which the mike is silently activated *without ringing* the phone. (Infinity miking works even with cell phones, so turn them off prior discussions.) If you're *really* concerned, then unplug the phone itself.

Poor Mr. Pen Register!   Poor Mr. Tap!

If you've followed my techniques, your home phone will have no revealing calls made or received. This will usually thwart the officials, as they rely on the pen register evidence to learn of one's associates and hopefully gain probable cause (PC) to obtain warrants (wire-tap, search, or arrest).

Even if they go ahead and place an illegal, unwarranted tap on your home phone (assuming they can discover it), you're smart enough (I would hope) to avoid hanging yourself with your own tongue. Apparently, there are some 3,000 words which trigger automatic recording devices--words regarding crimes, terrorist acts, wanted criminals, etc. Also, there is voice pattern recognition software which will automatically record any conversation with a suspect's voice. *Cuidado, muchacho.*

Red herring phone numbers

Many phone books today have reverse directories to look up a number or an address. Missing numbers are either non-working, nonpublished, or temporarily nonallocated. Find one which rings but is never answered, even late at night. That's "your" new number to give out, like the RR box number.

Voice mail providers are allotted a block of numbers, sometimes with a conspicuous exchange. These numbers are answered digitally, by computer. Clever folks have hacked into a provider's system and welcomed themselves to a number. Unless this number was assigned to a "real" customer, this borrowed number would likely go unnoticed for a while. If you do this, anonymously send the provider a M.O. for the proper fee when you're through with the number. Do not steal.

IN SUMMARY

Your goals are really quite simple: ❶ Not to draw attention to yourself, and ❷ To give investigators no place to go even if you *do* draw attention to yourself.

By having a phone number (VM#1) and street address (postal drop with no useful address on the application), by not acting like a drug courier or a Romanian spy, you've melted into the crowd. By not leaving revealing phone records on file, by not using the phones insensitively, you've nipped any remotely possible investigation of you in the bud.

You're enjoying the modern miracle of fiber-optic, satellite telecommunications without having it work against you. As I explained at the beginning of this chapter, using phones with discretion is the hardest part of one's overall privacy stance. **Beat the phones, and you're likely to win.**

It's a good idea to change phone numbers, code names/numbers, and calling habits often and unexpectedly. The Germans basically lost WWII because of lazy, overconfident communication habits.

Mix it up, stay alert, and *trust your feelings.* If you get an eerie read about something, *disengage immediately*--however inconvenient or costly. Then change your codes, tighten up your procedures, and lay low for a while. Correlate any new or unusual experience/person with your suspicions. If something/somebody is too good to be true, then it probably *is.*

"DIGITAL TELEPHONY"

At press time, the FBI has been seeking to grossly expand the *"Communications Assistance for Law Enforcement Act"* (CALEA). Although the drafters of CALEA explicitly stated that the statute was not designed to expand police surveillance, the FBI is insisting that every cell phone double as a tracking device providing instantaneous and continuous location of the user. Specifically, the FBI is demanding that the wireless networks be reconfigured and designed to facilitate:

● **Tracking of the physical location of a subject *any time a cell phone is turned on* (even if no call is being made or received), and subject movement *regardless of a carrier's service area.***

● **Delivery of this info to law enforcement in *real time.***

Currently stalled in Congress, FBI director Freeh and AG Janet "For-The-Kids" Reno have enlisted the public support of FBI agent James Kallstrom, chief "investigator" of the crash of TWA 800. (I say "investigator" because many witnesses have reported that a missile downed the aircraft. The Canadian military is said to have satellite photos of it. This is the cover-up of the decade. Our government is obscenely wicked.) The feds whine that murderous drug dealers remain uncaught because they reprogram their cell phones with new numbers up to 10 times a month, and there's no way to keep track. Stay tuned.

PRIVACY WITH PAGERS

A pager is a simple radio receiver tuned to a single frequency. Each pager has its own unique phone number. When called, the pager network sends out your page through all of its transmitters simultaneously (since pagers are passive and don't broadcast a *"Here I am!"* signal, as do cell phones). While your messages *can* be intercepted, your *location* can never be known through a pager.

Establishing service

The alphanumeric pagers require an operator to type in the outgoing message, which reduces your privacy. Therefore, I recommend a *numeric* pager, and buying it outright (they're only Ø80-110) to avoid a credit-based rental. You might have to pay a 3-6 month service deposit, which is no big deal. Don't flash a lot of cash, however. Mumble something about having to write a check--*"Oh, wait, I do have enough money."*

National paging services

If you travel often, or don't want your callers to know even your *general* location (through the area code and exchange), get service from SkyTel (800-362-5500) or Pagenet (800-PA-GENET). SkyTel is probably superior. You can choose portions of the country, or nationwide coverage. I recommend getting the voice mail, too. You have only a toll-free number and a PIN. It costs callers nothing, and they won't know where you are. Neither will SkyTel, until you call in to check your messages (always use pay phones).

If you don't ever want the provider to know your location, then skip the voice mail. Numerically, you'll have to be paged with codes, or callers can send messages through their computer to your *alphanumeric* pager (although plaintext messages are not private). Think it through first. I still think the voice mail route with numeric pager is best. You can have a friend in another state pick up your messages to confuse your location. **Tell your callers to *always* use pay phones and *never* leave their own phone numbers--codes only.**

The numeric Skypager Ultra is Ø99.95, monthly voice mail is Ø6.95 and service is Ø9.95-12.95 per month depending on how much you prepay (3, 6 or 12 months).

They'll want a phone number (use a local voice mail), an address (use a street mail drop), and credit card (tell them you prefer to send them a check, but send a M.O. for 6-12 months).

While reception is spotty in distant rural areas, all cities and busy highway corridors (i.e., S.A. to Austin) are covered.

Use a Personal Data Assistant (PDA)

All pager owners *must* buy a pocket electronic organizer (for Ø10-600) and password protect the names and numbers of your friends. **Names and numbers *absolutely cannot* be left on paper. There can be *no* excuses, *no* exceptions to this.** Once the information has been entered, *you must personally and immediately burn* the paper and thoroughly pulverize (or flush) the ashes. Do not simply throw away the paper, not even in some assumed "safe" place (out the window on the highway, in a public trash can, etc.).

"The kingdom was lost...for want of a nail..."

I'll give you an example how "half-assed" practices lost a war. It is now known that the Allies won WWII by cracking the U-boats' Enigma code machine. Ultimately, they did this by the mistake of only *one* German. The Enigma scrambled messages through use of several successive rotors. With the help of Polish exiles who smuggled out an early commercial model Enigma, the British cracked the 3-rotor machine. At last, the Allies could locate U-boats from their radioed position and hunt them down. U-boat losses then became immense; up to 40 per month.

Then, on 1 February 1942, the Kriegsmarine replaced the 3-rotor Enigma with an updated *4-rotor* version. "Shark" was 26 times harder to crack and could have taken years. Meanwhile, the U-boats became safe again and were starving Britain out of her shipments from America. If the atrocious shipping losses continued unabated for another 10-12 months, Britain would have been blockaded out of the war.

Finally, after nearly ten months, a miracle. On 24 November U-459 was shelled by a British destroyer. Damaged and sinking, the submariners abandoned ship. The captain's duty was to throw overboard the code books (on water-soluable paper) with the Enigma machine, but in the panic he forgot to do so. U-459 was boarded by two British sailors, Fasson and Grazier. Sadly, these brave men would go down with U-459 before escaping with the Enigma--though they *did* pass up the code books. The cryptanalysts were again (after 11 months) reading all U-boat traffic within weeks.

By war's end, the Allies were intercepting and reading German messages sent from the 100,000 Enigma machines-- often before the Germans themselves! Rommel (whose message traffic was compromised) often succeeded because he didn't always follow orders and thus didn't always move as the Allies had expected him! Though the German High Command broached the possibility of their messages being read, such was always dismissed as impossible because of "uncrackable" Enigma machine.

Without the failure of that U-boat commander, Britain would have been lost before "Shark" could be cracked by brute computing force. Without Britain as a launching pad, there could have been no Atlantic coast invasion or strategic bombing of Germany. The Germans, fighting a one-front war, would have pushed the Soviets past the Urals and had ample time to perfect their long-range bombers and rockets. The Allies would have been forced to negotiate a conditional peace. Had that U-boat commander tossed his stuff overboard, we'd be living in a very different world today.

The Allies "Ultra Secret" was kept until the 1970's, when the story was declassified. (Until then, our government sold captured Enigma machines to foreign governments without telling them that we could easily read their communications.)

The moral is: *Little* things can *indirectly* decide the *larger* matter. You simply *cannot allow* names, numbers and codes to fall into hostile hands. If threatened with arrest, it is *your* responsibility to utterly destroy your PDA. **You *cannot* fail that under *any* situation.**

Until your names/numbers can be stored/recalled in portable electronic form, they will have to remain on paper. This is obviously a very uncomfortable expedient. When on the road, they *must* be kept in a combination-lock briefcase *at all times*. A locked, closed container is immune from all intrusion except a PC-based search. Be prepared to burn your sheets if search/seizure is imminent. **Think in advance exactly *how* you would do this and *what* you'd need. Prepare *now*.**

General tips on using your pager

❶ **Keep a spare AA alkaline battery with you at all times.** At the "Lo Cell" message (after 3-5 months), you'll have a couple of days to replace the battery. Don't be left out because of a dead battery! Also, secure the battery cover lock.

❷ **Alter the sliding black switch** so that your pager can't accidentally be turned off, or into beep mode when tactics demand the silent vibrate mode. Simply heat a small knife blade and slice off the protruding portion of the switch. Well done, it won't deface the pager, yet still allow switchability.

❸ **In public, use the *vibrate* mode, for privacy.** Test it out on your style of carry to ensure that you can feel the sensation--which lasts for 5 seconds, and once every two minutes for any unread messages. Once at home or work where privacy is not a concern, switch over to beep.

❹ **If in a group, synchronize your pagers' time.** Accuracy is good for only 15-20 seconds per month, so you could be off by as much as six minutes per year. A commonly accurate timestamp might one day be very important.

❺ **"Sanitize" your pager by removing its phone number.** If lost, page it from a pay phone (or your public voice mail) and instruct the finder to return it for a reward.

Tips on calling back with privacy

❶ **If you have sensitive long-distance calls to make, *don't* call from home or work. Buy a prepaid phone card.** Use pay phones (which accept *incoming* calls) and have them ring you back if you'll be talking for more than several minutes.

❷ **Use pay phones!** I can't emphasize this strongly enough. It makes no sense for you and your people to be calling home-to-home when you have pagers. Page them instead, and they'll call you back from a pay phone. Keep a 35mm film can full of quarters with you.

While such secure operations may not be utterly necessary right now, they *will* be fairly soon. Even though a tap of your telephones is unlikely, it is easy enough to have a "pen register" placed on them. The snoops would then do a "C&A" (Customer and Address) search to know who and when you've called. The feds do this with suspected drug-dealers all the time (sometimes for *years* before the actual bust, to rake in as many in the network as possible).

Start a list of incoming-call pay phones and their location in your area, and compile them for your group. Eventually, when operational security becomes paramount, you'll need to make a coded list of these pay phones. Then, instead of leaving the actual # of the pay phone on your page, you'll leave the pay phone's *code* number (probably three digits) and the "pagee" will simply look up the code to learn the phone number (and location). The list should be kept (at minimum) in a PDA, and (at best) encrypted in a notebook.

❸ Once you've received a page, remember it or write it down, **and *erase* that page!** While your pager has a locked memory to store messages, don't use it. If found or confiscated, you *don't* want your pager containing stored messages.

❹ When returning a page, do *not* mention anything over the phone about getting a page. First of all, it's *unnecessary*; both of you *know* you got paged. Also, if a third-party is listening in somehow, he might learn about your use of pagers when he didn't know such before.

Using codes with your pager

With your compatriots, it's plain unadvisable to enter numbers in the raw. You'll need to encode certain messages.

The ✱ key and the digit block coding system

Fortunately, since the ✱ key (in most paging systems) acts as a space or hyphen, you can enter blocks of numbers of your own design. A simple, yet effective, manner of coding message is to use group info with certain digit blocks. For example,

Two digit blocks can mean messages,
Three digit blocks can mean locations and/or pay phones,

Four digit blocks can be the last four numbers (scrambled) of your people's phone/pager numbers,
Seven digit blocks (scrambled) are local phone numbers,
Eight digit blocks (scrambled) can be time/date (5:45 PM on 14 February would be, in the raw, 17451402), and
Ten digit blocks (scrambled) are long distance numbers.
I can't think any obvious uses for the 1, 5, 6, and 9 digit blocks, but you might. Within, for example, the two digit block, 00-09 can mean one group of messages (Go To...), 10-19 another (Danger Status), 20-29, and so on. Hash it out with your buddies and invent something clever, yet coherent. Don't outsmart yourselves and create a system *too* complicated to use.

Scrambling the 4, 7, 8, and 10 digit blocks with a key

If these blocks were sent raw, vital information could be gleaned from a page. (The 2 and 3 digit blocks, for example, are *already* coded listings and therefore do not need to be scrambled.) Therefore, you *must* scramble them. The simplest way to do this is to create a four digit "key" (which repeats when necessary for the 7, 8, and 10 digit blocks). For example, if you wanted your compatriot to call you at 555-1212 and your code key was 2468, simply add 2468246 (*individually*, digit by digit, *not* as whole numbers) to 5551212 to get 7919458.

2+4=**7** and 4+5=**9**, but how does 6+5=**1**? Simple: 6+5=**11**. To avoid creating an *extra* digit, just *ignore* the lefthand 1. (To decode, subtract 6 from 1 to get -5--meaning the integer 5.)

You don't add as *whole* numbers because you'll eventually get (with a high enough key and raw number) an *eight* digit block from a *seven* digit number (thus confusing the receiver into mistakenly reading it as an eight digit *time/date* block).

Never **write down the key.** Either memorize it, or enter it in your PDA as a $ figure somewhere.

This four digit key can easily be changed, and *should* be changed fairly often (at least every two months). Communicating a key change should be done only in *person,* and not over the phone, pager or mails. While a successive list *could* be used, if even *one* of your people were compromised--so would the list. (For example, *over half* of the Order's members ratted out their "kinsmen." Plan for this eventuality.)

In composing your key, do not use successive numbers (reverse or not, as in 7843) or any reuse of numbers (as in 7147). This will prevent any visual similarity between raw and scrambled numbers. One such break may be all somebody needs to crack your key if they suspected the raw number.

The message syntax

Since you are sending complex messages such as *"Don't go to our scheduled meeting place. Danger status now at Level 2. Member X has been compromised. Call me at 7#* (local phone) *at this 8# (time / date)."* Compose what you need to say and send it. The receiver will decode it and read it sequentially.

I recommend beginning your message with your identity (e.g., scrambling the last four digits of your phone number). Then, I'd signify the importance of the message--especially if you're instructing the receiver to call or meet you. He needs to understand the matter's priority so that he doesn't run to a pay phone for merely routine callbacks.

Sending long messages

Your pager's *screen* will likely hold a max of 12 digits (e.g., 313-555-1212). How *many* screens each message can contain depends on the paging company. Most systems will give you a second screen (though perhaps not all 12 digits as in the first screen). Therefore, a message can be at *least* 12 digits, and maybe 18, 20, 24 or even more. Whatever the capacity, it won't be enough for the really long messages. Therefore, one of your 2 digit codes should be *"This page is a continuation of the previous page."* so you can clearly daisy chain messages.

Keeping track of your clever messages

Obviously, you'll need to write them down, whether you're sending or receiving. Since you don't want to write them on paper, what to do? Go to an office supply store and buy a clear vinyl sleeve about 5"x7". On an insert card, graph out (as a template) how many blocks per screen your pager will hold. With a wipeable, colored overhead projector pen, compose (or decompose) your message.

Because of the structured insert card, messages are easily manipulated in proper order. Once done, spit on a tissue and wipe off the ink.

An even more secure code method

While the above scheme is probably good enough for most users, its ease of operation is a potential Achilles heel. The digit blocks are a giveaway to at least *some* kind of message syntax.

The ideal method, then, would be to have all your possible messages, locations, pay phones, etc. in a special software program, encrypted in your notebook. Let's say that there were 175 things for code number assignment. The program would, based on a key, assign these items a *random* number between 100 and 999. To change the code numbers, simply change the key and the program assigns new random numbers.

The program would also code/decode your messages *for* you. Enter the received page of "186-744-302" and the program would translate it as *"It's Bill. I'm running 30 minutes late. See you at the same place."* To send a message, highlight in order (from a menu of the 175 messages) what you want communicated and the program gives you the numerical string. It would even "know" when the message exceeds a page's digit capacity and daisy chain multiple pages to send. If your notebook had a soundcard and dialer, the program could even enter the page over the phone *for* you. Gee. Pretty neat, eh?

Where can you *get* this program? You can't--not yet. It's merely an idea of mine at this moment. If anybody out there wants to tackle this, I'd be happy to help with my input.

Why *bother* with this? Why not use PGPfone or Nautilus?

Encrypted, real-time phone calls have their place, no doubt. But encrypted analog cell calls *sound* encrypted and will get some attention quickly. While a strong encryption algorithm should thwart attack, that cell number will be fast pen registered, if nothing else. Your callers' and callees' phone numbers will then be a matter of record in some fed's file.

The great thing about pagers is that numbers sound like numbers (codes or raw phone numbers) and the owner's location is not trackable as is a cellular or landline phone.

Also, not everybody is able to *afford* notebook computers, encryption hardware, PC card modems and cell phones--*and* be proficient enough to use them. Thus, pagers are an affordable and *understandable* alternative that will serve surprisingly well with quality planning and discipline.

YOUR PRIVATE HOME

Your home should be a sanctuary; a dike holding back the vast ocean of humanity. With proper planning and discipline, its location will be an utter mystery to interested parties.

GOING PRIVATE FROM PUBLIC

Most of you are currently living in an informational fish bowl, totally visible to outsiders. Once your address is public knowledge, there's no making it private. You'll have to *move*. Correctly handled, a move cancels all ties to your old address.

Get your new place long *before* you need it

Remember Pascucci's hunt for the Nazi Koziy? Had he set up his second "flee-to" house *before* he needed it, his number wouldn't have been on the list of newly connected phones (or utilities). Arrange for your new home at least several weeks before moving so nobody can find it by some post-move activation date of phone, gas or electricity.

Buying a new place with privacy

This *can't* be accomplished in your own name. This also *can't* be accomplished through a mortgage. It will work *only* if you've the funds to buy a house outright, *and* if the house is purchased by an entity (which you control).

The entity

This is a trust or a corporation (Nevada, Wyoming or Delaware, which allow for *undisclosed* directors and stockholders). It has its own postal drop and voice mail. Your name should *not* appear as trustee, agent, etc. You discreetly move assets to the entity's bank account and have *it* buy the house, establish phone/utility connections, pay property taxes, etc. Under an alias, you can "rent" the place from your entity and pay with M.O.'s.

Not only is this utterly private, but you've separated ownership and control. Since there is peril to ownership, you want to merely *control* the asset. In a lawsuit, your house couldn't be taken away from you any more than your rental car. You just "live" there and pay rent, remember?

What about "allodial" titles?

An "allodium" was land given to Roman centurions, with title utterly free and clear of state encumbrance. All land in the U.S.A. *used* to be allodial. Part of the reason behind the Homestead acts was that the 160 acre parcels were allodial, and thus incapable of being stolen from the homesteader by scheming banks and speculators. Allodial land cannot be mortgaged or bonded against by government--therefore no property taxes, zoning restrictions or building codes apply. Allodial land is *your* land, utterly. We got tricked *out* of our allodial titles by the "fee simple" deed through the State.

While you can "re-allodialize" your land, it must be fully paid for and the process involves a public notice in your newspaper and notifying the tax assessor, etc. Obviously, not a very private process. I've *heard* that it works, that property taxes cease and the bureaucrats go away (after a long fight)--but I don't *personally* know of these success stories. Therefore, I cannot recommend the allodial position at this time, especially since it totally violates your locational privacy. However, I am willing to be convinced of any success story, so please write me if you've firsthand proof.

Renting a new place with privacy

It would be pointless to merely exchange one credit-checked apartment for another. You want to avoid giving out your SSN. Though difficult, it is not impossible to find places which will rent to you without a credit check or ID--I've done it all my life. In fact, I've *never* rented under my own name, nor have I been subjected to a credit check. (The secret is an honest face, lots of smiles and a hefty cash deposit.)

This is easiest in small college towns. Roommates are constantly needed, and if you don't look like a scumbag you're in with little ceremony. Cash deposits quench uncertainty.

...[A] *university is perhaps the best place in the world to lay low while establishing your new identity. The social climate is generally free and easy, jobs without strings attached are readily available, and the world in general doesn't make the kind of demanding requirements on college students that it expects of the average working stiff.*
-- Doug Richmond; *How To Disappear Completely*

If you've a family, then you probably don't want to share a place and you'll need a house or apartment to yourselves. This is most difficult still, and you'll probably need false ID as it's very unlikely (though not impossible) to be rented on your good looks alone--unless they know you or somebody who knows you. Farming communities are best. Trust is high there.

If you're heavily wanted, have a trusted friend rent a place *for* you. Pay your rent by mail and the landlord will never see you. If he drops by and asks where Fred the tenant is and asks who *you* are, reply that Fred is travelling and you're just watching the place for him. Smile and invite him in for coffee so that he can see you haven't trashed the place.

The utilities

Try to have the landlord handle this and reimburse him monthly. Explain that you can't afford the Ø50 new account fee, and offer to give him a cash deposit. I've done this all my life, too. (Once, I rented from Patriots who were glad to do this to help lower my exposure--but don't rely on such luck. I don't.)

If you landlord isn't keen on this (after all, there's nothing in it for him but extra hassle and risk), then all's not lost. You can, in smaller communities, obtain service without credit and ID. (By law, utilities must be provided, if for no other reason so that tenants don't freeze in the winter.) You'll just have to leave them a fat deposit. Pay your bills and go easy on the kwatts, or else the electric company will report you as a possible pot-grower using indoor lamps, and you *will* get a visit.

Your landlord

Pay your rent on time, *without fail*. **No excuses.** Sell your valuables if you have to, but *pay your rent*. Keep the noise down, and don't get the cops called on you. Avoid any domestic disturbances. Keep the place clean and tidy. Take care of the lawn. Show some pride your own appearance. Offer to make small repairs yourself, and give him the receipt. Tether your dog and keep him quiet. No wild parties.

Don't talk about radical politics, philosophies or religions. **Never talk about guns.** (If the subject comes up, say you had a .22 as a boy, but don't have guns now. This will appease everybody. Gun-owners will think you're still salvageable, and the gun-haters will praise you for "growing out of it.")

Before you sign your lease, firmly limit the "inspection rights" of the landlord. Insist on a change of locks (with full possession of *all* keys) and a 24 hour advance notice of any inspection (unless the place is flooding, on fire, etc.). Any presence of his outside the stipulated terms should constitute breaking and entering. You want your landlord to respect your privacy, and if he seems reluctant to do so during lease negotiations, find some other place.

I once rented a room in a friend's beach house. Since the place was constantly teeming with overnight guests and I was often travelling, I insisted on putting a lock on my bedroom door. I should have clarified this *before* moving in, but I didn't anticipate his unreasonable reaction. Even though he could have the spare key, he threw a *fit*. He insisted that *his* overnight guests shouldn't be *"forced to sleep on the floor when there's an unused bed in the house."* He called me *"unsociable and paranoid"* and just couldn't understand why I didn't want strangers in my room and in my bed. (A semblance of rationality eventually prevailed, though not without strain on the friendship. I soon moved out.) Moral: work all this out *first.*

The timing of your move

Unless you want to simply be followed from your old job to your new place, you should (suddenly, without notice, if you think you're under surveillance) quit your job the day *after* your "public" move. In my chapter *Earning A Quiet Living*, I'll get into more detail. A job, unless paid in cash, is never private because of SSN tracking. You should have your own cash economy business.

You shouldn't move *during* scrutiny, but months *prior.* While it can be difficult to know just *when* you will come to the attention of somebody, guess earlier than later.

The moving sequence

Here's how it's done, in eight easy steps.

❶ **Establish a *temporary* voice mail number (VM#1).**

This is the number you'll give to real estate agents and prospective landlords. You don't want *any* of their calls going to your old home number or its replacement voice mail number. **Remember, *no links* between the old and the new.** While still at your old place, do not create any local call MUD's to this VM, your new home number or landlord. Use pay-phones.

Tell the VM provider and real estate agents that you've just moved in town and are looking for a place, so your mailing address is General Delivery. If they express any suspicion, say that you're staying with friends and you don't want to bother them with your mail and phone calls.

Once you've at last moved in, this VM number will have served its purpose and you should then cancel it.

❷ **Get a P.O. box for your *private* correspondence.**

Never use this for anything but receiving letters from friends, or else it'll quickly get on a mailing list owned by TRW, etc.

Receive at your *new* home any mail which is unavoidably *directly* related there (utilities, phone, property taxes, etc.). See, if the electric company *already* knows your *home's* location, then why inform them of your P.O. box, too? (*Never* provide additional information if you don't *have* to.) Also, if your P.O. box is ever monitored, your home's location won't be indirectly discovered through the electric company.

❸ **Establish a permanent voice mail number (VM#2).**

Get it from a different voice mail provider, using your new P.O. box or G.D. This will become your new number for *trusted* friends. They will be instructed *never* to give out this number. If you're under severe scrutiny, have them call you from pay phones and avoid creating MUD's on their home number.

❹ **Change your "official" address to a *street* mail drop.**

This is done weeks before moving. Have *all* your official and business mail rerouted there. Change your license and registration, credit cards, library card, voter's registration, checks, etc. Filing a postal change of address form goes a *long* way in creating the desired false trail, as it's provided to over 70 direct mail marketers.

For ultra-privacy, get the mail drop in another city nearby enough to service once a month or so.

However, the most cursory of investigations will reveal your "home" address to be merely a mail drop. So, either use my RR box ploy, or:

> *Set up a "legal" address somewhere else, such as a closet at a friend's house, containing some misleading personal effects (books on* [benign] *subjects you have no interest in, and clothes a few sizes away from your own). He can thus point to something if ever questioned; but, of course, he hasn't the slightest notion when you'll be returning from India...*
> *-- 100 Way To Disappear and Live Free;* Eden Press

❺ **Establish VM #3. Drop your old home number.**

This is also done at *least* several weeks before moving, and from a totally different provider. Get all your acquaintances, "mere" friends and public used to it. This number will serve as a calling buffer to hide the timing of your move. Otherwise, your home line being suddenly disconnected would send an *"I've just moved"* message to anybody who called. Check messages from pay phones only, *not* from your new home.

You will *not* be able to change your home number to the voice mail number through the phone company. The voice mail provider leases a block of numbers from the phone company, so the phone company cannot therefore deal directly with you.

❻ **Do *not* hire a mover. *Gradually* do it yourself.**
Do *not* have a "moving" sale or make announcements.

The logic of this should be obvious. You *don't* want your neighbors to know that you're moving. If possible, move from an enclosed garage over a period of several weeks--the last trip being a couple of months before your disappearance date. Well done, you simply evaporated and your old neighbors never knew you *had* moved out--much less *when.*

Your neighbors probably cannot help but notice a trip or two, however, so you'll have to yarn them with *"some stuff is going in storage"* or whatever.

If you must sell some stuff before your move, do so *weeks* before disguised as a *yard* sale. Do not have a yard sale at your new place, as some unwanted person is bound to show up.

Since you will be living in your old place for weeks *after* your unknown move (to maintain the *appearance* of normal residency), leave a car load of necessities there. Once you're leaving for the *last* time, scour the place (especially the trash) for *anything* which might enlighten an investigator. Unwanted stuff you should drop off at the Salvation Army or Goodwill.

Don't alienate your old neighbors. Return any borrowed items and make good on any promised favors. Once they discover that you've actually *moved*, they'll be at least a little hurt if not downright pissed-off, so you want to have in advance ameliorated as much bad feeling as possible. If you need help to move, pick some trusted *best* friends. Throw a nice party or dinner for them afterwards. Instruct them that your new place is to be private.

❼ Leave some false leads.
If you think it's clever to leave utterly *no* leads, then think again. By leaving *no* leads, you'll frustrate and fascinate the investigator and make him *really* sink his teeth into your case. You don't want your case to become his Cause.

Your false leads should be *shrewd*. The more *subtle* the better. Weeks *before* moving, create a MUD to a local travel agent. Go visit her and explain that you are moving to San Diego and ask for info. From your old home, make a few phone calls to the San Diego Chamber of Commerce and receive some brochures. Mention to your mailman, gossipy friends and neighbors that you've always loved San Diego--but say nothing about *moving*. Establish a mailbox there and have your nontrusted people write you after you've split and done ❽.

Don't make your misinfo ridiculous. Don't spread the word that you're moving to Alaska when it's common knowledge that you hate cold weather. Keep the B.S. plausible.

The more time an investigator spends on false leads which have been "confirmed" from several angles, the less time he can spend on *real* leads. Digging through your trash, he already found a bookstore receipt for *Guide to San Diego*, so he's hooked. If you keep your misinfo subtle and let *him* make the links between your bogus triggers, he'll *stay* on the false trail. (Remember, he's not accustomed to anybody as *smart* as you who's using a book as *good* as this.) As more and more time passes, the case becomes more and more stale. Assuming that you're no great crime figure, and that you haven't personally pissed him off, your case will be quickly back-burnered.

❽ After some months, cancel VM#3--your "official" number.
Keep this VM number only if need it for "public" or "legal" reasons (job, classified ads, etc.). Remember, you should be dropping many people from your life. Since privacy measures complicate things, you must simultaneously whittle down your social sphere. *"Three can keep a secret if two are dead."*

Your method of "social triage" is up to you. You'll be somewhat amazed (and hurt) at the small number of your "friends" who actually miss you and make any *real* effort to keep in touch. If you're not appreciated once gone, then you probably weren't very appreciated when around. Ghost out, and the social fluff won't really notice. ***Nothing personal--it's just the way most people are these days.*** If they ask, reply that you've *"been travelling"* and *"we'll get together soon."* That'll hold most of them. Tell the pushy ones that you're in-between places and just staying with friends for now.

In review

Your business/official mail gets shunted to a street addressed postal drop, which has only an RR box#. The buffer VM has only that postal drop address. Your old phone number has no linking MUD's or long-distance records to your new place. Your trusted friends have a separate channel to call and write you, and even if they *are* pen registered, all that can be learned is VM#2 and its P.O. box. Big deal.

The only way you could be found is if you or a trusted friend were actually *followed* to your new place. But to be followed *to*, one must first be followed *from*. Anybody under such intense, expensive surveillance should move out of town (if not the state), drop *all* previous contacts and not return to regular haunts (bars, restaurants, dry cleaners, grocery stores etc.) Examine your cancelled checks and credit card records to learn what these old haunts are--*he* will. Don't have magazines, newspapers and mail orders sent to your new place.

Think things through, use wisdom in which friends you trust and lay low for a while. The feeling of new freedom and personal control will prove incredibly refreshing.

ONCE AT YOUR NEW PLACE

Drop all old spending habits.

Don't use the same: pest control, delivery or security service, housekeeper, yardboy, etc. Don't update newspaper or magazine subscriptions; buy them at the newsstand. (The traitorous Christopher Boyce--"The Falconer"--was caught by resubscribing to a falconing magazine from his Oregon hideout.) I'd even change hairstylists. Go through your cancelled checks and credit card records and list all the past businesses you must now avoid. (I repeat this for emphasis.) It should *appear* as though you've moved overseas, even though you maybe only moved just across town.

Modify or drop all past associations.

Be *very* careful about which friends and relatives know your new address and number. Trust me on this: if your privacy measures are tight, then an investigator will focus on finding you from your friends and family--either by interview or surveillance. Pen registering their phone lines is an easy way to find you. Have them call your national 800 pager from a pay phone, and return their call there by prepaid calling card. If the feds are *really* serious about you, even *this* wouldn't be safe enough, in my opinion. Cease communications entirely.

Don't blow it by getting all paranoid

O.K., so you've made a slick move and regained the privacy of your domicile. Don't stupidly draw attention to yourself by being overtly covert. The best example of this is a Duluth guy known to every UPS deliveryman as "The Hand." Whenever "The Hand" receives a parcel to be signed for, a mere hand darts from a cracked doorway for the clipboard, signs it within the bowels of his house and returns it, by hand only. Although his face has never been seen, he's *blown* his privacy. I don't personally know "The Hand." I heard about him only *third*-hand (ha, ha--pun unavoidable). **Moral: suspicious activity *will* get you talked about far and wide.** Don't be *too* cagey with your new neighbors.

Appear lower middle-class. Keep a low profile.

Barry Reid wisely recommends not living in a place more expensive than the average cop can afford. Anything more expensive paints a big *Sue Me!--Raid Me!* target on your head.

Pay your rent, don't alienate your neighbors and keep your mouth shut. Keep your shades drawn. Don't be effusive, either. Don't show them your guns or books. Don't discuss politics or religion, however tempting. *Never* carry your actual address on you or in your car.

Don't take in boarders, renters, or casual guests.

While you may like the rental income, the sacrifice of your privacy probably isn't worth Ø350 a month. Such people will pick up all sorts of useful information on your habits and plans.

Remember, at least 80% of those you know will roll over on you with enough carrot or stick. (For a real landlord scare, watch *Pacific Heights* with Michael Keaton.)

Handy Boston tip: If you *truly* need to give somebody a house or padlock key, make successive copies of it, which by the 3rd or 4th generation will not work. Give out the *penultimate* copy, which is an inadequate master from which to make copies.

Hidden caches

There are many books on this subject. Have a "fall guy" safe with a bit of cash, benign diskettes, and valuables to satisfy any raid or burglary, while your extremely well-hidden floor safe goes untouched. Great caching locations include ceiling beams, electrical outlets, doors, bookcases, stairways and ceilings. Use imagination and quality carpentry. (Small fire-resistant lockboxes start at Ø20. Use them for cash and valuable papers.) Bury some of your stuff on and off your property.

Watch your trash. *Burn,* don't throw away sensitive stuff.

Be very scrupulous about this. I throw away nothing which has names, handwriting, or addresses on it. In fact, I burn nearly all printed and packaging material, receipts, etc. All anybody would learn by going through *my* trash is what kind of breakfast cereal I eat. If you can't burn in town, lock away the papers in a briefcase and drive to the country.

Dealing with unwanted persons at your door.

Never allow salesmen, religious doorknockers, etc. inside. Even a casual glance inside your home can be educational, and investigators are very good at posing as innocuous passersby. Speak to these people only through the door or intercom. If an emergency is claimed, offer to make a phone call *for* them, but do not allow them inside. (If you need convincing on this point, watch *A Clockwork Orange*--otherwise *avoid* that movie.)

In the year 2000, your neighborhood will be swarming with "Fed For A Week" census takers. The census has been perverted into an obscene decennial snooping where dozens of personal questions are demanded of you. (Gee, how did the U.S. Army *know* exactly *where* the 140,000 Japanese-Americans were, in order to cart them off to desert tarpaper shacks? From the 1940 census.) "Explain" you're just housesitting for the owner, or that the place is currently unoccupied and you're cleaning it up. Regarding the mailed questionnaire, not returning it will get you a personal visit--so, fill it in with B.S.

Store your extra stuff

Do not keep all your worldly goods at your new place, even if it's roomy enough. Spread your eggs out into at least a couple of baskets. That way, if your house is cleaned out (by fire, flood, theft, or seizure), you can still start over. **Never have *all* of your cash, books, guns, vehicles and trade tools at home.**

A motor-home or travel trailer parked in the country

This the best choice, in my opinion. While independently mobile, RV's are much more expensive and less roomy. Some prefer the modularity of a tow rig and trailer.

Stock it for self-sufficiency with tools, books, food, guns, clothes, cash, gold/silver coins etc. Set it up in the country on some old couple's farm for Ø50-100 a month, or in exchange for helping them out. Not only have you solved your storage needs, but you've created an inexpensive retreat to go to for vacations or in times of trouble. For shoestring budgets, order *Travel-Trailer Homesteading Under $5,000* from Loompanics. (Although I wouldn't want to *live* like author Kelling, such makes for a great cheap retreat.)

Rigs shorter than 24' are really too cramped, and those longer than 30' are a real pain to drive or tow (requiring a heavy-duty tow rig). Buy something at least five years old (for good value) and post-1982 for good style and function. Although you can get lucky and find a Ø4,000 cream puff, expect to pay up to Ø6-9,000 for a decent one. Pressurize the water system for 24 hours and carefully check for leaks. Buy it under an alias different from your rental alias. If you won't drive or tow it very often, don't bother registering it--it's more private and saves Ø.

I have lived and vacationed in my motor-home for years. I've even written one of my books in it. Mine has hundreds of books, a good stereo, CD's, breadmaker, TV and VCR with lots of movies, electric piano, computer and laser printer, reloading equipment, toaster, blender, juicer, dehydrator, and lots of stored food/water. They can be comfortable to near luxury. Within their limitations, they're pretty neat. Being cute and cozy, your date will even think it's romantic.

They make great guest homes for your out-of-town friends. You could even have several RV's salted about the country in your favorite places. You'll have no hotel bills, less packing and the safer geographical diversity of your stuff.

Or, it could serve totally as your "Mr. Hyde" place. Your home is squeaky clean, while the RV contains your "subversive hate" material, books, guns, reloading equipment, etc.

Storage units

I don't care for them. They're expensive and get broken into fairly often. However, if the RV route isn't for you, or if you've got too much furniture, you'll have to rent a unit.

Since any tenant-landlord face-to-face is probably only during the rental, have a friend rent it for you. Your name won't be on the lease and the manager will never have seen you.

Pick a place with a security gate, as this dramatically cuts down on the petty burglaries. Usually, there will be a 6 or 12 month deal, and you should go for it. It's cheaper, and there's less of a paper trail than by paying monthly. Pay by mail with M.O.'s from another town.

For your "home" address, do not give your public mail drop, and do not give your P.O. box. Use a one-time apartment or hotel address (without mentioning any room number). They'd only use the address to notice you of the auction of your stuff for unpaid rent, anyway.

You might find somebody willing to rent out their *garage* for storage space. This alternative is cheaper and more private, though not as safe as a security-gated storage facility.

Keep utterly *no* records or receipts of the unit at home. Hide them in the unit itself, or someplace nearby. If transported in your car, keep them in a locked briefcase.

BOSTON T. PARTY THOUGHTS

Let's face it: if you're not at least a *plausible* annoyance to the draconian forces, if you don't bang your head against the rules, if you don't have some assets and personal freedom on the line--*then what good are you?* The human capacity for obedience probably borders on the infinite, but how often is such obedience deserved by *government?* Quit worrying about your precious stuff, take some quality precautions and give 'em hell! We may indeed suffer a 21st century Dark Age in America, but by God, let's at least make them *earn* it.

Be a barnacle for Liberty, and slow down the ship of Tyranny. If there are enough of us barnacles, then perhaps we'll eat through the hull.

❖ 14

PRIVACY & YOUR GUNS

(2000 Note: *Boston on Guns & Courage* is essential reading!)

THE PURCHASE

Buying privately

In probably 20 or so states Americans can still privately buy and sell firearms without any forms, paperwork or registration. In many cities there is a classified ad section for guns (if not under "Guns" or "Firearms" then often under "Sporting Goods"). Call from a pay phone and pay cash.

Or, go to a gun show and seek out the private sale tables (they'll usually advertise this with a little sign). At gun shows, beware of anybody suggesting that you participate in any unlawful activity, such as "straw sales" (buying a gun on behalf of somebody forbidden to do so themselves). If this happens, it's probably a BATF agent trying to set you up. Threaten to alert the police if he persists. BATman or not, he'll leave at once.

The FFL

If you buy or sell through a federal firearm licensee (FFL), then you must fill out a Form 4473. These forms are, illegally, being photocopied or scanned by BATF agents for the growing national database. Avoid FFL's if at all possible. At least use the RR box trick for your address--that's vital.

OWNERSHIP

First rule: *Keep your mouth shut.* Do *not* tell your neighbors, landlord, acquaintances or casual friends that you own any guns (much less what kind and how many). When Confiscation Day comes (and it *will* come), there will be toll-free fink lines. Will Americans snitch on fellow Americans? Count on it. They'll see it as their civic duty as law-abiding citizens. The Ø1,000 reward won't hurt, either.

Fugitive-from-injustice Gordon Kahl was ratted out by a daughter of his hosts. For Ø25,000. The feds crept up on Kahl from behind and shot him in the head. (Kahl was sitting in a chair, watching TV with the volume way up, as he was hard of hearing.) When the sheriff blanched at that, the feds shot *him* and blamed it on Kahl. They then chopped off Kahl's hands and feet with an ax, then doused the place with fuel to hide the evidence. (The concrete structure didn't burn down, and a reporter later found a foot under the fridge.) In a privately funded exhumation and autopsy, famed L.A. coroner Thomas Noguchi confirmed that the foot had indeed been intentionally severed and the body purposely set ablaze between two mattresses. Any skeptics of this should order the documentary video *Death and Taxes* from retired Phoenix officer Jack McLamb's *Police Against the New World Order* (602-237-2533).

Moral: Reward money *works*. Keep your mouth shut.

Record and hide your guns' serial numbers.

Have a data sheet for *each* gun to prove ownership if necessary. *Never* make a *list* of your guns--one sheet per gun only.

The concealed carry permit

Some 28 states have now passed CCW's or liberalized their laws to Florida-style *"shall issue."* While this no doubt resulted *in part* from public pressure and the political efforts of Gun Owners of America (GOA) *et al*, I'm still somewhat skeptical. Now, the government knows the identity of several million Americans who have the *temerity* to actually *bear* arms.

I firmly believe that gun ownership and gun bearing will eventually be outlawed through a U.N. convention on "Gun Trafficking" or "Disarmament." **Such a U.N. convention will *constitutionally* overturn these state CCW permits.** Naturally, it will be challenged in court (as was the Brady bill) and will probably be upheld (as was the Brady bill). It is good to recall that registrations invariably lead to outright confiscation. Ask the British, the Canadians, and now, the Australians.

So, before you run out and get your permit, think long and hard about the possible consequences down the road. Do you *really* want to be fingerprinted and pay Ø50 per year for something that is your *right*--only to suffer confiscation five years hence?

I won't do it. Self-defense is my right, and I won't beg for permission to exercise that right. I'll keep my name off the master list and carry privately, thank you. I'd rather be tried by twelve than be carried by six, as it's much easier for my family to get me out of jail than the cemetery. Congress recognizes *"Refuseniks"* like me, so they passed H.R. 3610 (*The Gun Free School Zone Act of 1996*) to herd us into the safe corral of CCW's.

Carrying discreetly without a permit

In open carry states, no permit is required. However, open carry not only compromises your privacy, but you risk unknowingly passing within 1,000' of some school two blocks away and committing a federal felony! H.R. 3610 has all but *killed* open carry rights--rights normally untouchable by the feds--and is the beginning of the final onslaught of gunowners.

So, how to carry *de facto* concealed without a permit? Usually, a gun in its *"holster"* is not considered to be *"concealed."* A holster doesn't necessarily have to be the classic leather hip holster. The SafePacker from Dillon Press (800-762-3845) is a square Cordura *"holster"* (by judicial agreement, I understand) which resembles a cell phone case. Gun fanny packs and gun purses can stretch the legal definition of *"holsters"* so check it out in your state.

If you don't live in an open-carry state, and want to conceal carry without a permit, you'll have to technically break the law. Boo, hoo. The only ways you'd be found out are if you were frisked, or if you had to defend yourself. The odds on either are pretty remote. A behind-the-back holster underneath a vest or jacket works well. Shoulder holsters print obviously, and gun fanny packs are too well-known. Ankle holsters are cumbersome, create a limp, and hold only small pistols. Gun attache bags are fairly indiscreet. For *deep* concealment, use something like ThunderWear which holds your pistol inside the front of your pants.

Buying accessories

Do so at gun shows with cash. Or, alias order COD from a pay phone and pick up your package at a mail receiving service. Don't *subscribe* to gun magazines. Don't buy gun related stuff by check or credit card. Ideally, there should be absolutely *nothing* on paper to indicate that you're a gun owner.

Storing your guns privately

At home, keep only what you *need* for self-defense. You won't need your full arsenal to stop a burglar, and your full arsenal won't stop the federal ninja. (Besides, they're going to confiscate what they find in your house anyway, so keep the rest elsewhere.) No more than one pistol and/or one rifle or shotgun per person at home is necessary.

If you have more than that (and you *should*), store them elsewhere *not* under your real name. I wouldn't *bury* them unless you *really* know what you're doing. Underground caching has its place, but don't go crazy. You want most of your guns *accessible*. Digging up cached guns and cleaning them up takes a lot of time. Would you bury your only fire extinguisher?

Shooting your guns privately

The gun club and range

I would *support,* but not join, your local gun club. Have a friend tell you the combination to the gate, or go with him as his guest--but do *not* join the roster. Send them an anonymous M.O. for the dues, *but stay off of their list.* Gun club members will one day be rounded up for questioning and home searches.

On public land

Done sparingly and in varied locations, this isn't a problem. Keep the sessions short and lock up your guns, ammo, brass, gear, etc. in the *trunk* before you go. Have nothing in your interior's plain view to even suggest that you're a shooter.

On private land

There are two trains of thought on this. The first is: Don't draw attention to yourself and alert your neighbors to your gun ownership. The other is: Damn it, it's *my* land, I can shoot on it legally, and I *want* the neighbors to know that we're armed. I can sympathize with both.

Some of my neighbors have been shooters, while others were not. I guess it all depends on where you live and who's around. One thing I would *never* do is fire fully-automatic weapons on private land--not even the perfectly legal "Hellfire" devices (which sound just like fully-automatic fire). This will likely alarm even your gun owning neighbors, and the Sarah Brady's will certainly call the feds.

SELLING YOUR GUNS

In a word, *don't*. I'd sell a kidney before I sold off my guns. Guns should not be merely a hobby or some form of recreation. Guns are *"liberty's teeth"* (George Washington) and to sell off the teeth is to guarantee your future slavery. It is the 2nd-Amendment which protects the other nine. Keep your guns.

If you *have* to sell a gun or two to streamline your battery, then get an *ad hoc* voice mail number just for the classified ad. Pick up your messages and return calls from a pay phone only! Meet the buyer in a discreet place (e.g., a gun store parking lot where gun handling is normal) and accept only cash. It is illegal to sell to out-of-state buyers, minors, convicted felons, fugitives, and those under the influence of drugs. Do not break any laws.

TRACKING OWNERSHIP

The trail ends with the first private sale wherein no state or federal paperwork is made. Such private sales exist primarily in the South and the West. If you sell or pawn a gun to an FFL, a receipt must be filled out. To get that gun back, you must fill out a Form 4473--even if you bought the gun privately.

Avoid having to fill out the Form 4473. I know people who have dozens of guns, all purchased privately with cash. There's not a scrap of paper, not a cancelled check, not a charge card record, not a magazine subscription, not a CCW permit--*nothing* to indicate that they are vociferous gun owners. This situation terrifies the government. There are more guns in America than Americans. The feds will *never* find them all. Tee, hee.

THE COMING GUN GRAB

I'm not worried about a successful gun confiscation program in America. I just don't know if enough Americans will have the guts to shoot government thugs. *That* is the only relevant question regarding future gun control. On this point, I quote from a speech by the late novelist Taylor Caldwell:

I hate to throw a somber bombshell into this festive gathering of patriotic people of good will, but life is too short to be sweet. With the matter of catastrophe facing our county, we have a terrible alternative now. We actually have two alternatives. We can say: "Hail, Caesar, we who are about to die salute you." Or we can say what

Quincy said in the first Congress: **"One day we free men will have to exit. It is inevitable but whosever, whenever, or however we go down, we'll exit as free men."**

I'm going to castigate all you men here for what you have to America--every mother's son of you.

How did we arrive at this disastrous hour in time? I will tell you. **You men...abdicated your manhood!** *You deserted the Republic. Aristotle said two thousand and five hundred years ago:* **"Masculine republics decline into feminine democracies and democracies into despotism."** *That is what has happened to America now. We call ourselves a free country. We are not free! Tomorrow the tyranny will be overt instead of covert as it is now.*

...Now, above all, you men have--what is the phrase--you've "chickened out" out on your women and thrown them into confusion and terror. I've listened to some of you men who have defended yourself to me. We want peace and tranquility, men say. This will never be a peaceful and tranquil world until the last human being is dead. We are made that way. And all the Sunday school teachers and nice nellies and psychiatrists will never change that. **They are trying to make us all sweet and docile so we will offer no resistance to despotism.** *(This brilliant observation is also the premise for Ira Levin's dystopic novel* This Perfect Day. *BTP)*

Is there any hope? Well, only a little, and I'm afraid that few men will take advantage of it. **One:** *Challenge your government and, if you suffer for it, to hell with sweet peace.* **Two: Fight gun control!** *It is your right to bear arms under the Constitution but the tyrants want to take away your arms so you won't be able to offer any resistance to bayonets!*

Gentlemen, you can restore your dead Republic. But be again the masters of your government and be again the masters of your women or will you meekly say: "Hail, Caeser, we who are about to die salute you."

Don't worry that they'll get your guns. Worry that *you* might not have the *guts* to use them. Will you let federal barbarians storm your neighborhood, breaking down doors--or will everybody on your block rain a torrent of copper-jacketed lead on these thugs? It's about to hit fan--will you be courageous?

If *you* can't imagine--gasp!--defending *your* rights and *your* property and *your* family against the Government, then sell your guns to a *real* man. Who are you fooling--you don't deserve a Zeiss-scoped Sako any more than a .22 Jennings. Give up your guns now and spare yourself the embarrassment later. **The 2nd Amendment is for *men*--not hobbyists.**

A QUIET LIVING

*With five notable exceptions, nearly everyone in our society works at a job of some kind and is automatically suspect...if he doesn't work. The exempt classifications: The very rich, who obviously don't need to bother working, the very poor, who also don't need to work because the Welfare State takes care of them. Then housewives, students and retirees. Everyone else in the U.S. and Canada is expected to work **or at least have the appearance of working**.*
   -- Doug Richmond; *How To Disappear Completely* (1986)

Much has changed since 1986. A *sixth* exemption should now be added: the home-based entrepreneur, which I discuss later in this chapter. Although ideal privacy is attained through one's own small business, not everyone is, or can be, an entrepreneur.

PRIVACY ON THE JOB

   Most people work for a company. I will show you how to increase your job privacy, although jobsites are not private because of SSN tracking. Also, your employer can spy on you:

Once you are hired, there is virtually no limit to the information your employer can [legally] gather. He may listen to your telephone conversations, monitor your keystrokes on a computer terminal, and even ask your neighbors to describe your habits at home. If you [claim] worker's comp..., he may place your name in a computerized database that other employers may consult when they are making hiring decisions. He may even hire informants to spy on you.
   -- Mark Nestmann; *How To Achieve Personal & Financial Privacy In A Public Age*, Fifth Ed. (1993), p. 91

Filling out the application

To avoid suspicion, you *must* have what *appears* to be a street address and home phone. Unless you are to go through a security background check for job clearance, your "official" address street mail drop and voice mail will serve just fine.

Your work time line must not contain any curious gaps which imply periods of unemployment. While references are rarely checked, make sure that yours do not contain any great triggers to your current domicile, activities, etc. Any particularly nosey questions should be answered N/A (not applicable).

For SSN, I'd leave it blank *until* you are hired. Once you are hired and on the job, *then* you should spring any untax posture on your new employer. Even if you *do* allow SS and "income" tax withholding from your untaxable private-sector remuneration, there's no reason to sprinkle about your SSN to every *prospective* employer.

Beware of any waivers of personal privacy which you might be asked to sign. These would include submission to drug tests (which are often inaccurate) and polygraphs (which actually measure stress, and not prevarication). There are often state and federal restrictions on use of the "whiz quiz" and "the box." Also, companies *so* suspicious might not be worth it. How much you are comfortable with signing away is up to you.

If, by the time you are reading this, some form of national ID workers' card has been instituted, avoid getting one at all costs. Instead, show the prospective employer your records of birth, or passport. If unacceptable, start your own business-- but refuse to get a federal cattle brand!

The job interview

Don't act weird or covert. Seem personable and outgoing-- you *like* people. You are *sociable*, not a hermit. It does not enhance your privacy for it to be *known* that you savor your privacy. Also, show moderate excitement to be working for them, and express a desire to make it your "home."

On the job behavior

Have no illusions: your email and phone calls are easily (and legally) monitored by your company. Be discreet. Also, many companies prohibit firearms, so conceal *well*.

Your new coworkers

They will naturally want to get to know you. Do not shy at having dinner or drinks if invited. Do not discuss politics, religion or philosophy. Do not rail against the government any more than the general level of discontent. Do not admit that you own any guns, even if your coworkers do. Trust somebody only if you *can* and if you *need* to.

> ...[A]*void giving background information to fellow workers. If you're planning to stay...only a short while, however, make an effort to plant false and misleading information in the minds of the other workers, such as your favorite pastimes, places you'd like to travel or live someday, and your plans for the future. Insulate your private self by keeping your personal interests and ideas to yourself alone.* **Share the spurious with the curious.**
>
> -- *100 Ways To Disappear and Live Free*; Eden Press, p. 14

Leaving employment

The odds are that you won't be working for Wonka Widgets for the rest of your days, and that you'll eventually leave--or be fired. The general rule is to *leave on good terms*.

How to quit

They'll *know* why you're quitting--no Hamletonian soliloquy is necessary. Be gracious and act with style. Give them fair notice (usually 2-4 weeks). Train your replacement well. Make them sorry to see you go, even if you were kind of a pain. Don't leave bad feelings behind which can fester into lies.

What if I'm fired?

Same rules apply--be gracious. *"But I was 'discriminated' against!"* **Yeah, so *what*?** Can you refuse to marry somebody based on their race, creed, color, religion, "sexual orientation," economic status, education, or personal hygiene? Certainly! People "discriminate" (show bias) every day against others. **Only government hasn't any right to "discriminate" because it exists by us all, for us all.**

So, why don't private *companies* deserve the same right? Because the Supreme Court says it *"affects interstate commerce."* So what, you got fired. Just because not everyone on the planet *likes* you, don't be a big baby and file an EEOC suit. Even if you sincerely believe you were fired for being a left-handed Lithuanian lesbian, *drop it.* Find a company *owned* by left-handed Lithuanian lesbians and go work for *them*.

START YOUR OWN BUSINESS

By the year 2020 "Self" will be the largest employer. Such is *the* key to not only financial privacy, but to financial success. Wealth comes from profit and capital gains, *not* salaries.

What *form* of business?

I tried a partnership years ago, and they're like a marriage. While they *can* work, be cautious of whom you get involved with and write down a comprehensive agreement on duties, responsibilities, etc. Beware of the "mutual agency" of partnerships; each of you is liable for the debt and obligations incurred by the other. Finally, partnerships rarely end on pleasant terms--so, your privacy can be deeply compromised.

Corporations and trusts have their place, but learning enough about them may be too demanding at first. Begin with a sole-proprietorship *in your own name* and avoid having to file a DBA (doing business as) form.

What *kind* of business?

Whatever we do for money is usually oriented towards:
People (sales, health care, hairstylist, therapy, etc.)
Information (computer programming, research, etc.)
Things (car mechanic, inventor, construction, etc.)
I recommend that you develop marketable skills in *each* of the three areas. For example, an individual competent in tutoring, bookkeeping, and locksmithing could grow a successful business *anywhere* in the country. There is safety in diversity.

Not everybody, however, can be such a generalist. If, for example, you are *not* a "people-person" or mechanically inclined, then only the Information field is open to you. So, if you are clearly attracted to a single area, try to develop several marketable skills *within* your area. Being a plumber is fine, but learn how to fix cars and computers, too.

Whatever it is, *do what you love doing*. That's the only *real* "secret" to success. If you're not doing--*right now*--what you'd *rather* be doing, then change it--*right now*. Probably 90% of people die with deep regret how their lives "went"--and they generally had no excuse for it but themselves. Live *your* life.

The main thing to remember

Your eternal enemies will be Envy and Greed. These are personified by bureaucrats, gossipers, thieves, and moochers. They share a dilemma which complicates the lives of cannibals: no reuseable victims. They're always looking for a new meal.

Be private. *Don't...*

get an Employer Identification Number (EIN) or DBA.
hire employees.
allow "public access" to your home.
get a business phone unless the Yellow Page ad is vital.
get a business bank account.
don't get a business or professional license.
charge or collect sales tax..
advertise too publicly.
attract attention of the bureaucrats.
let disputes sour into lawsuits, formal complaints, etc.
accept checks, if possible.
offer receipts--make them ask for theirs.
declare this *"remuneration"* as taxable *"income"*.
keep your expense receipts at home--hide them if kept.
don't brag about your success or speak of your affairs.
ever admit that your engaged in a *"trade or business"*.

Be private. *Do...*

insist on cash, or *postal* M.O.'s (cashable at any P.O.)
offer prompt, quality service and honor your word, *always*
quietly operate under your own name--avoid "retail" sales
pay your independent contractors in cash
get a separate voice mail number for business calls
get a separate P.O. box or mail drop for business letters
appear *moderately* successful, but not wealthy

Consider a mail-order business

It has little or no local visibility, therefore the city, county, and state bureaucrats will probably never notice you. Also, it's very low-key financially (no 1099's filed on you), so the IRS will probably never notice you, either. Receiving cash and M.O.'s (which you can either cash or endorse to make them bearer instruments) creates far less records than depositing checks at a bank. Also, cash and M.O.'s do not bounce like checks do.

Almost *anything* can be (and is) sold by mail. There are forums available for any product, especially on the Internet. Payment comes in; product goes out--simple and quiet. You can (and probably should) operate out of your house. Work in a suit, or in your underwear--it's your choice. If you're painfully shy or just plain ugly, who'd know? Customers like your ad and buy your product. You never have to see or talk to them! For privacy and flexibility, nothing beats mail-order in my experience.

THE PRIVATE CAR

It is amazing the number of people who take their cars with them when they disappear. When they do, it makes the Missing Persons Bureau's job so very, very easy. All they have to do is wait until the current license or registration expires, then get their information from the renewal or switch. Whether you sell it, swap it or ditch it, your car will be a very valuable and readily discovered clue to your new location and identity.
-- Doug Richmond; *How to Disappear Completely*, p. 39

Vehicular privacy depends on: how you buy and sell it; how you register it; and how you drive/park it.

PURCHASING YOUR CAR

If at all possible, you should purchase your car with cash. Most private sellers will appreciate cash. Dealers, however, are not so keen on it. If the amount is over Ø3,000, a dealer (though not private seller) is supposed to report the transaction with a CTR to be cheerfully filled by yourself. Simply purchase several postal money orders (M.O.'s). They're available up to Ø700. You do not have to produce ID during their purchase. Be careful that you do not engage in "structuring."

Another reason to not buy from a dealer is that they usually won't help you reduce sales tax by writing up a lower price. Private sellers, however, are delighted to help. (I've bought dozens of vehicles throughout my life and only *once* did a seller refuse this. He was a crusty Olde Pharte. I walked away from the deal. You should have heard him sputter.)

If your assets are considerable, then you should own your rolling stock through entities (corporations, trusts,

Unincorporated Business Organizations, foundations, etc.) These entities may hold bank accounts and tender checks.

REGISTERING YOUR CAR

First of all, try to get the seller to simply sign off the title, omitting a date. Explain that you'll probably resell the car soon, or that you're not sure exactly how you'll register it since the car may go in your new company. Write up a single bill of sale for yourself, which you keep. Most sellers will have no problem with this--they just want your money and to be rid of the car.

The advantage of a signed title is that you can sell the car without first having to register it yourself. The car is still in the seller's name, and after many months he won't remember your name if asked. You can probably get away with renewing the plate tags as the registered owner, though you might have to show "proof" of insurance (which is easily created on any home computer). Just don't cause the seller any problem by racking up unpaid parking tickets or robbing banks. I've bought many cars this way, kept them for up to 3 years and sold them without a problem. My name was never affiliated with those cars. Pretty ghostly, eh?

Some states (i.e., Washington) thwart this practice by requiring the seller to fill out a detachable sales invoice and sending it in the DMV. Know the peculiarities of your state. You won't be able to pull this off forever, so keep sharp.

If you have to register your car

There are many Sovereign Right-To-Travel plates running around, and while I admire the daily courage and tenacity of these folks, such isn't for me. *Technically,* they're right--a car is a private conveyance free of all licensing requirements, and a *"motor vehicle"* is operated in commercial capacity, thus subject to registration and regulation. Unrequired registration turns a car into a regulated *"motor vehicle."*

Practically speaking it's a weekly hassle. Impoundment is common, and I've yet to hear of *anyone* getting their car back through even the best legal arguments. (State Citizen Extraordinaire Richard McDonald simply uses reliable, old BMW's from the wrecking yard for their relatively painless confiscatability.) The *"vehicle"* vs. car battle will *someday* be won, however, it's not *my* battle. I use motorized conveyances to *enhance*--not impede--my travel.

So, to travel around without hassle, you'll need some form of government-issued plate. Simple reality. **Never register a car in your *own* name**--use an *entity* (trust, corporation, etc.) as your "heat shield." Make sure the address is a dead end. I hear that Tennessee doesn't require insurance or smog tests.

Foreign plates

Even better is to "foreign flag" (as are airplanes and oil tankers) your cars in another country. Establish a foreign entity, have it own your cars, and get foreign plates. I could explain exactly how to do, but you should earn it. Besides, if *everybody* started driving around with Madagascar plates the whole concept would be ruined by saturation. There are companies selling registration and plates from the Turks and Caicos and the "Washitaw Nation" (see 7/6). Use extreme caution here. *Your* butt is on the line, so check it out thoroughly and talk to those who've used it *successfully*.

Whatever you do, make sure that it's all legitimate and that the paperwork will withstand a 30 minute computer check. Have your bill of sale handy. A *really* suspicious cop will simply impound the car and tell you to hash it out with the judge. So, be on solid ground and have a convincing story why you're on the road with yellow Dutch license plates. (Speaking with a Dutch accent would be enormously helpful.)

USING YOUR CAR PRIVATELY

As I say repeatedly, *don't draw attention to yourself.* Don't drive like a maniac, don't have glaring equipment faults, and don't park it inconsiderately. Having an understated econobox, Ford Taurus, or OldsmoBuick wagon helps to lower your profile. Unless obviously a work van, vans attract the cops. You might want to even remove identifying stickers and nomenclature for that extra generic look. Back in to conceal your rear plate. Use an enclosed garage, if possible. Pay off parking tickets--or better yet, feed the meter and don't get parking tickets. Avoid valet parking.

If you're mechanically minded, do your *own* repair work to avoid exposure at the dealership. Buy the parts with cash, from different stores. Don't become a regular at the local NAPA. If it requires a professional mechanic, choose a small independent garage over a dealer if you can. Remove all interesting items and use an alias for the work order. Pay in cash, obviously.

Stuff to have in your car

Inside the passenger compartment, and within a *locked* bag, I would have: binoculars, scanner, and ham radio. Keep an overnight bag on the rear seat (with clothes and toiletries) to pose as a traveler, if need be. For any paid tickets, have copies of the M.O. and certified mail. This will effectively rebut the *prima facie* evidence of an erroneous FTA warrant. Have your driving paperwork *handy* (not in glovebox) to show a cop.

Inside the trunk, I'd have 5 gallons of water, tools, car parts (belts, hoses, plugs and wires, cap and rotor, drain plug, oil, coolant, etc.), and backpack filled with end-of-the-world gear (pistol, jacket, hiking boots, hunting knife, tent, bag, etc.).

For only Ø155, you can buy two great rifles (a .303 Lee-Enfield No. 4 Mk.I for Ø85, and a .22 Marlin 60 for Ø70) and store them unloaded together, with ammo, in one Ø25 case. The .303 cartridge (available at any WalMart, etc.) is 90% as powerful as the venerable 30-06 and the Lee-Enfield has a detachable 10-round box magazine. It's quite powerful, reliable, and accurate. I can hit a Bad Guy-sized target at 400 yards from standing with a tree rest. If stolen or confiscated, you're out a whopping Ø85. (There's even an Indian .308 Winchester variant of the Lee, but I wouldn't trust the quality.) Have the Lee cut down to carbine length with an 19" barrel, and remove the extraneous wood. The .22 Marlin is a fine little rifle, especially for Ø70. Find both at any gun show.

But hey, if you want to trunk your Valmet and scoped .308, go right ahead, but you're taking a bit of a risk.

A cool Boston tip on counter-rousting gear

A foolproof way for the cops to create probable cause (PC) is to have a drug-sniffing dog "alert" to drug scent planted on your trunk lid. How does the dog handler plant the scent? By touching a twig of pot in his pocket and wiping the scent on your car. It's guaranteed PC on demand. I know; it happened to *me*.

My countermeasure: Make the dog *terrified* of your car. How? With the **Dazer** from U.S. Cavalry (888-888-7228; stock

#N9539; Ø34.95 plus Ø7.95 s&h). I thought of this idea while writing *You & The Police!*, but couldn't find the equipment.

[This ultrasonic dog deterrent is a] *high-tech alternative to chemical sprays or physical violence. A 2-3 second burst or quick on/off action deliver a discomforting yet humane, high-frequency sound inaudible to humans.* **Aggressive dogs become dazed or confused and retreat to a safe distance. Effective up to 15' away.** *Includes a long-life 9V battery. Measures 2"x4½". Weight: 3 ozs.*

During a detention you will not be permitted to hide your hands, much less hold the Dazer. So, you will have to mount it in your car. To hardwire it, buy a 12V to 9V power jack for cigarette lighters (KMart, Radio Shack, etc. sell them for Ø8. Keep the 9V battery as backup). I'd replace the Dazer's internal switch with a switch/oscillating relay hidden under your dash or in your glovebox. (The oscillation turns the Dazer rapidly on and off for best effect.) The Dazer itself (or at least its speaker) should be mounted under the car, probably pointing at the ground. (Left inside the car it might not be loud enough.)

I'd activate the Dazer whenever you are on the public roads or parking lots. That way, your car is protected while you're inside a store, etc. Also, you might not have the opportunity during a traffic stop if detained outside your car.

If you properly refuse consent to a search of your locked trunk or car, the cop will often call for a drug dog. Then the fun begins, but *do* try to keep a straight face. Immediately tell the K-9 to *"Back off!"* He won't get *near* your car. In fact, he'll want only to run to the squad car and cower on the back seat.

The cops will be extremely baffled and disturbed by this. "Explain" that you've always had a "way" with animals and that they obey you. No sniff, no alert, no PC, no search.

Do *try* to keep a straight face.

SELLING YOUR CAR

If you need to dump your car, sell it yourself to a private party for cash. Be careful not to reveal anything to this person about your real plans or reasons for selling. He would be an ideal source of information...for snoopers, thanks to the efficiency of auto registration systems throughout the country. **The buyer will, of course, be an excellent place to dump your <u>fake</u> information...**

-- *100 Ways to Disappear and Live Free*; Eden Press

If the car is registered in your own name, set up an *ad hoc* voice mail number for the classified ad. Meet the buyer somewhere public. Be honest about the car's condition and mechanical history--don't lie to him. Price your car fairly, with slight room for negotiation (but not too much, say 10-15%).

Politely insist on cash. Explain that you don't have time to wait in line at the bank. Offer to leave the sale amount on the title blank and he can fill in a lower amount to reduce the thieving sales tax. Nearly all buyers will appreciate that. Once, I sold a car to a company and since they wanted to record the *full* purchase price (deductible as a business expense), my offer had no leverage. Also, they insisted on paying by check for the paper trail. Since I needed the money and there were no other prospective buyers on the horizon, I took the check.

PRIVATE TRAVEL

It's becoming more and more difficult to travel *incognito*, but it *can* be done and I'll show you how.

THE BUS

Nobody travels by bus in America because they *want* to. I would almost ride a bicycle than ride the bus. DEA and INS agents patrol the bus stations like hungry sharks. Your travelling companions will seem from another planet. A long-distance bus is more often than not a rolling bad neighborhood, and the ride is a working definition of eternity. Sorry to be such a snob, but is saving a few bucks over a flight really *worth* it?

RENTAL CARS

You'll need a credit card and driver's license. While you can pay with cash once the car is returned, your credit card voucher will be meanwhile kept on file until then. If the voucher is made through the *electronic* card reader, then the card company will know of your location and car rental.

For maximum privacy, have a friend rent the car for you. Drivers over 25 y/o may use another's rental car.

Some rental companies sticker their cars. The ones in Florida no longer do after enough foreign tourists got carjacked and killed. The reason carjackers preyed on rental car drivers is because they were likely from at least out-of-state, if not overseas, and therefore would *not* be one of 340,000 Floridians with a lawfully concealed pistol. (That's something Dan Rather didn't tell you about...)

TRAVEL IN YOUR CAR

Much of this was covered in Chapter 16, *The Private Car.* Pay for gas with cash--do *not* use credit cards (one of Ted Bundy's many tactical errors). Do not drive at indiscreet speeds. I wear a touristy T-shirt of the area so I'll look like Joe Roadtrip if stopped. Have all sensitive stuff in the trunk.

If you travel with a pistol, keep it in an unlatched combination-lock briefcase on the front seat. If stopped, quickly unload it, put the mag and ammo in the glove box, lock your pistol in the briefcase, and the pistol is no longer *"on or about your person."* (This tip from my *You & The Police!*) If asked if you have a gun in the car, say no and that guns *"frighten"* you. Refuse consent to *any* search. (Got a *Dazer* in your car?)

DOMESTIC HOTELS

While motels generally don't ask for ID, most *hotels* do. Where you stay is up to up. Don't make *any* calls directly from your room--*no exceptions!* If it's a *really* sensitive call, don't use the pay phones in or even near the hotel.

A paid room is considered a *"house"* for warrant requirements. Don't open your door to the police; speak to them *through* the door. Don't allow officers inside without a warrant. Don't get the cops called on you in the first place.

DOMESTIC AIR TRAVEL

Ever since the Unabomber's threat to down a 727 out of LAX in spring 1995, passengers have been obliged to show ID during check-in. This was *supposed* to be, of course, "temporary" just like the WWII 5% "Victory Tax" on wages. This kind of crap is never temporary; it's merely the latest click of the tightening ratchet. Get used to it, for now.

Don't despair--Boston is here for you. Remember my little saying about government tyranny: *The tighter the net, the more slowly it must be trolled through the public ocean.* The bright, quick little fish have always escaped, and always will.

Buying your tickets

First rule: *never* buy your tickets at the counter with cash. This is typical behavior of drug couriers (who imagine they're being really sneaky). Many airline tickets agents will alert the airport DEA office, in hope of a reward. (America is the land of the snitch.) Instead, go to any travel agency, arrange your flight and pay for your tickets with cash.

At the agency, do not balk about providing a phone number or address--you should have *already* established your postal drop and voice mail (as I outlined earlier). **Remember, you'll be expected to have ID matching the ticket name.** Once you get proficient at the ID game, reserve some ID just for air tickets and alternate their use. Fly under one name, rent a car under a second, and hotel check-in under a third.

With the travel agent, be polite and *moderately* friendly, but do not get too chummy. If asked a personal question, *lie with the truth*. Spin a yarn with something you know. If you say "Baltimore" without ever having been there, it'll be your bad luck if she grew up there and wants to reminisce.

Exactly this happened to the *In The Line Of Fire* assassin. Opening a bank account under an alias, the clerk asked where he went to school. He replied that he attended New Brighton in Minneapolis. Being from Minneapolis, she immediately became suspicious as she *knew* there was no "New Brighton." Realizing his mistake, the assassin tried to smooth it over with, *"You know, you have a very pleasant way about you."* (which I thought was a very slick line to a lonely, overweight, bland woman). Later he showed up at her house, killed her and the roommate to cover up his blunder. His overreaction provided the loose end Clint Eastwood needed to unravel the case.

I realize that good travel agents are hard to find, but use different agencies from various cities. You don't have to buy your tickets in the same city you're flying from.

The demise of the travel agency

Soon we will reserve and ticket our *own* flights on the Internet and the travel agency will only plan package trips. TA commissions were limited in 1995 and it now costs them Ø28 to issue a ticket--so, it's not worth it for the cheaper flights.

What this all means for privacy is unclear. We might soon be required to key in our DNA ID number with every reservation, or some similar B.S. I'm glad that I got most of my travel done years ago, when it was much more free. For example, you *used* to be able to fly on somebody *else's* ticket--no more.

I'd get a private plane and avoid the travel hassles, whether by commercial air or by road.

Packing your bags

This should be done with great forethought, especially if you fly with a firearm. In Chapter 11 of my *You & The Police!* I explain how to do this. Unloaded, case locked, declared firearms may be lawfully transported in checked luggage (unless prohibited by your destination, like NYC).

Sensitive items and papers should be in locked in a hard pistol case with little combination locks, and the case locked in a checked bag. *Really* sensitive papers should be in a stamped, addressed Priority Mail pouch, and the pouch in your carry-on bag. They can separately X-ray the pouch, but cannot open it without a postal inspector with probable cause.

It is suspicious *not* to have tags on your baggage. Use the kind, however, which cannot be publicly read. Your address should match the one (if any) you gave the travel agent.

What to wear

Your goal is to be comfortable, yet not draw attention to yourself. Americans are the poorest dressed passengers in the world, so if you dress down a bit you'll fit right in. A good wardrobe is chino-type slacks and a simple button-down shirt. It's informal, comfortable, yet has at least a *bit* of style. Avoid flashy shirts, hand-tooled leather boots and expensive jewelry. Ladies, if you'll dress up a bit you'll be less bothered by officials.

Don't travel with excess keys, pocket change, etc., and avoid metal-laden clothing, especially belts. I've got a good friend from Austria who loves western clothes. After visiting me in Texas and buying Wrangler snap-down shirts, a silver necklace and bracelet, and a spectacular concho belt, he took off for the Orient. His clothes must have had three pounds of metal in them, and he had to practically undress at each metal detector. Just unlooping and relooping his concho belt took several minutes in itself. He was some frazzled by the time he got to Singapore, via Tokyo and Hong Kong.

Make sure that you've removed all telling personal items from your wallet and pockets, such as business cards, lists, etc. Carry a microcassette recorder with blank tape for any confrontation with airport cops. (If you don't tape the Scene, they'll claim that you cconsented to a search.)

Checking in

Your goal is to get your boarding pass and check your bags without being remembered. Get there early enough to avoid looking harried, and have your stuff ready (bags tagged, ticket ready, etc.) Do not act furtive. You're on vacation and you're happy, remember? You're merely a grain of passenger sand on an airport beach. Request a forward, window seat. You'll exit the plane more quickly and you can unobtrusively doze against the bulkhead. (I use foam earplugs and sleep perfectly.)

I don't like my baggage claim stubs stapled to my ticket, preferring instead to carry them in my wallet for privacy's sake. After getting your ticket, discreetly remove the stubs.

Going through security

Do not go to the bathroom directly before or after clearing security. Such is done by drug couriers who are constantly adjusting the parcels taped to their bodies. You shouldn't be smuggling anything, so don't worry about it. The only exception is if you're carrying a lot of cash. Post-1990 bills have a platinum-on-polyester strip which can set off detectors, so remove those strips. Carry the cash *on* you, and not in your bags.

Do not be surly with the security staff. Be polite and don't complain if they want to poke through your bag. Open it with cheer and assure them that they're just doing their job.

Airport behavior

Enroute to your gate, just do what everybody else does. If in a hurry, jog. If you've plenty of time, casually make your way, stopping at the gift shop.

I advise against making *any* phone calls, however innocuous. Airport pay phones are routinely pen registered and even monitored at the direction of a surveilling agent. You should have made your calls beforehand. Your pickup party should know to check your flight number in case it's running late, so you won't be expected to call him.

I prefer to get to my gate straightaway, sit down and read. When I say read, I don't mean just turn the pages--I mean *read.* If you've caught some agent's attention, he will look you over with binoculars across the terminal from behind a mirrored window. He will scrutinize your eye movements, and spot any nervous hand/foot movements. Therefore, pick a seat which is not easily observed, sit down and *read.*

If you need to use the bathroom, by all means do so--but only *once.* Repeated trips to the bathroom are typical of drug couriers. Do not make frequent trips to the water fountain--such implies nervousness.

If accosted by airport security or DEA, they will demand to see your tickets and ID. You are under no legal obligation to comply. Start your tape-recorder. **You should *never* go where *"we can talk more privately."*** Stay put--make a scene if you have to. Demand to see and scrutinize their credentials--write it down. (If they refuse, express disbelief that they are truly officers or agents, and thus powerless to detain you. *Then* they'll show you their badges.) **Keep asking if you are free to go.** If they claim *"reasonable suspicion"* to detain your luggage and it contains something politically incorrect, state your possessory right to it (so that they can't claim you abandoned it) and excuse yourself to get your lawyer. Leave the airport *immediately.* You should have already read my *You & The Police!*

On-board behavior

If there's ever an example of how *not* to behave during a flight, this is it:

> In October [1995], Gerald Finneran, described as one of the leading authorities on Latin American debt, was arrested at JFK airport in New York as he disembarked from a United Airlines flight from Buenos Aires. According to passengers and crew, he had lost his temper when flight attendants refused to serve him more liquor, assaulted them, **defecated on a serving cart,** cleaned himself with the airline's first-class linens, and thus left an odor that remained in the cabin for the remaining four hours of the flight. (BTP note: From Buenos Aires to Malos Aires. Here comes the best part.) *(The flight could not be routinely rerouted to land sooner because one of Finneran's seat neighbors was the President of Portugal, and flights*

containing heads of state are harder to divert.) (Surely we're
approaching the end of civilization... BTP)
-- from *News of the Weird*

His client fined Ø5,000, the attorney for "Exlax" whined,
"Maybe the skies aren't so friendly anymore." I know Ø5,000 is a
stiff, but Finneran got his money's worth. I mean, what would
you pay to assault flight attendants and crap on a serving cart
beside the President of *Portugal?* Ø5,000 seems a *bargain*.

I once called a flight attendant *"Darling"* and farted next
to a Guatemalan Air Force colonel and was fined *Ø4,000!* Just
think what a mere Ø1,000 *extra* would have bought me. (That's
what I get for not reading the brochure.)

Anyway, once aboard you're home free, *if* you can possibly
manage to restrain yourself from crapping on the serving cart. I
realize this is infeasible for leading authorities on Latin
American debt, but do *try*.

Picking up your bags

Go to baggage claim without delay. At some airports,
baggage handling is so efficient that it sometimes beats the
passengers. Get there before somebody walks off with it, as
stub verification by airport personnel is almost nonexistent.

Pick up your bags, and *leave*. Airports are hazardous
environments, full of federal agents, drug couriers, terrorists
and leading authorities on Latin American debt. I prefer my
party to pick me up *outside* baggage claim and therefore not
have to park. You should have arranged this before your flight
and not need to call them upon arrival.

Also, I prefer to dropped off at the curb and not have them
come in with me. I like a simple, clean *Bon voyage* on the
outside, so I can concentrate on making my flight. Also, my
attention is fully torqued up, scanning the boarding gate crowd
for anybody remotely resembling a leading authority on Latin
American debt who cannot help but soil my flight's serving cart.

INTERNATIONAL FLIGHTS

Many of the same tips for domestic flights apply here.

Your passport

Only one American in six currently has a passport. Apply for yours today. It's no big deal. First-timers must apply in person (at any substantial Post Office) with a notarized copy of their birth certificate and photo ID. Other than demanding a street address and your SSN, the form's questions aren't terribly intrusive. (Use your "public" mail-drop street address.) Leave unanswered any *"optional"* blocks. Notate that you'd like the 48 page passport (as the standard 24 pages fill up quickly). I recommend using *older* photos of yourself, especially for renewal applications (which are simply mailed in). Why keep the feds up to date on your current visage?

Your passport will arrive in 4-8 weeks. Photocopy the bio page and secure with your other valuable papers. Notice the bar code on the inside rear cover. Until they start putting bar codes on our hands, the passports must suffice.

Buying your tickets

Your ID will be more carefully checked at the international airport, so don't book under an alias unless you can back it up. Get a direct flight if possible. From major hubs as Dallas, Chicago, Atlanta, L.A., etc. one can nonstop to nearly anywhere. Don't describe your travel plans, just get your flight. For maximum privacy, get a window seat and sleep.

Packing

Go easy on the clothes, especially the shoes. Pack one change of clothes and a toothbrush in your carry-on bag, in case your checked luggage is delayed or lost. Hard bags with rollers are incredibly convenient for long airport hikes, and hold up better from indifferent foreign baggage handling. Collapsible luggage carts are, to me, more trouble than they're worth. Be a big spender and rent an airport cart for Ø1.50--or hire a porter.

Buy a neck wallet before you go, and carry your passport, traveler's checks, VISA and photos of your travelling companions (in case they become missing, so the police will have their photo). Wear that neck wallet *everywhere*--without exception. In your bags, have copies of your passport and the traveler's checks receipts (don't carry them with the checks).

Bring some interesting trinkets from home to give as gifts to your hosts. A small photo album will show foreign friends what your American life is like. For the flight, carry drinking water and a small spray bottle to spritz yourself.

What *not* to take

Leave your Uzi and C-4 at home. (Besides, you can buy them in any country.) Make sure no stray ammo cartridges are left in your luggage or pockets. Purge any local or sensitive paperwork, receipts, business cards, etc.

If you're taking a notebook beware that encryption software (e.g., PGP diskettes) and hardware (e.g., security PCMCIA cards) are considered *"munitions"* by the feds and forbidden to export. While few notebooks are really scrutinized and the Department of State recognizes a *"personal use exemption"*--beware. **Personally, I'd *never* leave the house with raw data on my notebook.** Encrypt your hard disk (also containing PGP software) with a PCMCIA encryption card disguised by false label as a RAM flash card.

What to wear

Dress in quality casual clothes. For myself, I prefer to wear a suit and tie and fly Business or First Class. I've never had problems. Officials generally don't mess with wealthy businessmen. (Once, I was even asked if I was a diplomat!)

Check-in

Get there *way* early. Relax and act excited about your trip. If you schmooze the ticket agent about this being your very first flight on TransOcean Airlines, she might even upgrade you to Business or First Class for *free*.

During the flight

Discreetly inquire if a Gerald Finneran is on-board.

Clearing foreign Customs and Immigration

They are primarily concerned if you have enough traveling funds to avoid becoming a welfare case in their marvelous Socialist country. For young people, having a gold VISA or American Express card goes a long way in smoothening your way. (And leave your ratty jeans at home, please.)

If asked where you'll be staying, mention an upscale hotel. (If you're *really* serious about your cover story, then you should have already made reservations there, in case they check.)

If you're visiting Israel or some other sensitive country, ask that your passport *not* be stamped, or at least a stamped paper be merely stapled inside. This is a fairly common request.

Staying in foreign hotels

The desk clerk will invariably want to see your passport, if not photocopy it--if not keep it during your stay. Do not allow this. Explain that you took it to the Fulmarian Consulate for a visa. Show/give them a photocopy instead.

Do not let the hotel hold your room key while about town. You don't want the front desk knowing precisely when you come and go. If your key is generic (without the hotel's name), then keep it on your person. If not, then hide it somewhere in the hotel, or nearby. I devised a clever way to hide mine, but I can't tell anybody--not even *you*. Sorry.

Be nice to the hotel maids

Leave a Ø2-5 tip every morning for your maid. My mother convinced me of this, calling it inexpensive theft insurance. Neither of us have ever suffered pilfery by the housekeeping staff. Even if you're only staying one night, leave a tip. It's thoughtful, *and* you might leave something in a room one day. Which maid is likely to turn it in--a tipped or untipped?

Above all, be kind to the hotel maids. They are neither subhuman nor second-class people. They perform a thankless, menial chore for messy, snotty guests.

Don't be the haughty American. Here's what happened to one such guest in Mexico. A heavy partier with his buddies, he treated the hotel maids with unconcealed disdain. Nevertheless, they were unfailingly polite and cheerful to him-- especially on his *last* day. After returning home, he understood *why*. Developing his vacation film, he noticed an unfamiliar photo which he didn't take. One maid took a picture of the other. With our hero's toothbrush. Only the handle could be seen. Proudly protruding from her big, fat, slightly out-of-focus *butt*. Revenge is a dish best served *cold*...

Be *nice* to the hotel maids.

Getting around overseas

Planes, trains and automobiles. Europe, for example, is so compact that air travel isn't really necessary. Take the train. Forget Eurail passes; they force you to stay on the move to get your money's worth. Simply buy your ticket and step aboard.

The *MitFahrGelegenheit (MFG)*

The *MFG* is a neat thing. In German it means "passenger opportunity." *MFG* agencies are in nearly every town across Europe and will (for a fee of Ø3-12, depending on trip distance) put you together with a driver going your way. With gasoline being Ø3.50 per gallon, most Europeans can't afford to drive alone for long distances. So, a driver calls up the agency and says that he's going to Munich on the 8th and has room for 2 passengers. He pays no fee to the agency. The passengers pay the agency's fee, and an agreed maximum of roughly 5¢ per mile to the driver. The agency won't ask for your ID. Reserve your *MFG* by phone, drop by, pay the fee, get the driver's name, call him and arrange the price and pickup. The driver doesn't have to know your real name or your address. I prefer to be picked up outside the train station. If you don't care for the driver, the agency will make another introduction for you without charge.

I've used *MFG*'s many times, without a hitch. I made some good friends, and never did the drivers charge me the full rate. I've ridden with all kinds of folks, from student musicians to an army captain. The *MFG* experience is faster, cheaper and more personable than the train. You might have to wait a couple of days to find a tricky route, but you'll always be able to get close enough to take a short train ride. Take along some fruit to share or a guitar to play, relax and enjoy your trip.

Returning home and clearing U.S. Customs

This is a real joy. I think that some of our federal officials are now being trained by the *SicherheitsDienst*. I once returned home through Atlanta, and DEA was there to greet our plane, all suited up in black ninja gear. Barking at us to stand in line and place our bags to the left, our bags were sniffed by two drug dogs. There was no *"Good afternoon, ladies and gentlemen. We are drug enforcement agents and this spot-check is purely routine. We apologize for this delay and welcome you to the United States."* Rather, it was like getting off the train at

Auschwitz. It was an utterly embarrassing and disgusting display of naked power.

Treasury Enforcement Communications System (TECS II)
The first checkpoint will be the TECS II counter where your passport will be scanned. If you are wanted in the NCIC, suspected/convicted of smuggling, drug dealing, or tax evasion, or wanted for jumping bail you will be detained at the very least. If you are snagged here, remain silent, reserve your rights and state that you wish to speak to your attorney.

Clearing U.S. Customs
I prefer to declare nothing and go through the green lane. Focus on the person ahead of you, and walk straight through without glancing at the agents to your side. Flit your eyes about and they'll call you over for a baggage search.
If snagged anyway, don't raise a fuss. Coolly cooperate. Avoid bringing back certain furs and leathers, ivory, etc. and you'll have no surprises. Also, you're supposed report over Ø10,000 in *"cash"* (cash, bearer notes and bonds, blank or endorsed checks and M.O.'s, etc.), so know that in advance. If they find unreported cash in excess of Ø10,000, it *will* be confiscated and you'll be arrested. It's nice to live in such a free country.

Leaving the airport
If you were hassled by the feds or the airport police, do *not* use the pay phones. You should have already arranged for your ride home. If things were really dicey clearing customs, or even if you just have an eerie feeling, beware. The authorities may already have probable cause on you and are waiting for you to charitably lead them to the friend picking you up, or to your car in airport parking. Wave off your ride with a covert signal (e.g., scratching your nose) and take a cab to some prearranged meeting point (e.g., a mall, etc.). Similarly, do not walk to your parked car. Take a cab and come back later for your car.

❖ 18

PRIVATE ENTITIES

You must begin to cultivate a change of thinking regarding business structures. Sole proprietorships and partnerships leave the owners vulnerable to business risk. What you must do is to *separate ownership from control* to create a legal posture of limited liability. While corporations can accomplish this, they offer little privacy in exchange for increased regulatory hassles (unless chartered in Nevada, Wyoming, or Delaware).

TRUSTS

Trusts are the common-law antecedents to modern corporations. Not only is ownership separated from control and your privacy protected, but trusts can lower your taxes.

Tax avoidance is *legal*. Tax evasion is *illegal*.

Tax evasion is like walking out on your dinner bill. Tax *avoidance* is using a free-dinner coupon to legally avoid paying. Or, say there were two bridges next to each other--free and toll. To sneak across the toll bridge without paying is evasion, but it's legal avoidance to use the free bridge.

The only thing is...the road to the *free* bridge is uphill, inconvenient and obscure, and the bridge itself is long, dark, narrow, and seemingly rickety. Conversely, the road to the *toll* bridge is a downhill highway and the bridge is short, wide, well-lit and secure--*everybody* seems to be using it! And they are... What they don't realize is that it eventually leads to a *cliff*.

There is nothing illegal or immoral about using your constitutional rights and statutory loopholes to minimize (or even eliminate) your tax burden. There is no obligation to pay one penny more in taxes than the legal requirement.

What is a trust?

A trust is a contract whereby A (the **Trustor**--the one who *trusts*) entrusts the ownership of his property to B (the **Trustee**--the one who is trus*ted*) to manage on A's behalf. Parents, for example, act as trustees for their children's funds. Since your right to contract for lawful purposes is unlimited, a trust is perfectly legal if there is no fraud or mental incompetence involved. Trusts may be revocable or irrevocable.

For tax purposes, the less power the Trustor has over the Trustee's management and disposition of the trust assets, the better. In short, the less control the Trustor has, the more unassailable the trust. When the Trustor has too much direct control of the trust, the courts may disallow the trust as a separate entity because **a Trustor *cannot* be his *own* Trustee.**

What's in it for the Trustor?

The Trustor has merely nonvoting Certificates of Beneficial Interest (CBI's--similar to corporate nonvoting common stock) which he can sell or redeem when the trust is liquidated.

So, the Trustor exchanges his assets for these CBI's and holds on to them tax-free while the trust's net worth grows. Once he sells the CBI's for cash, then the capital gain is *de jure* taxable--but we live also in a *de facto* world. In order for capital gains to be taxed, the IRS must first *know* about them. If the CBI's are sold out of the country and the proceeds transferred to the Trustor's *foreign* bank account, who is the wiser? This, however, would be construed as tax *evasion*.

Since we want tax avoidance and not tax evasion, the Trustor should *borrow* against his CBI's. **A collateralized loan is *not* a sale and the funds received are *not* income.** The Trustee has a foreign investment entity for just this purpose--to be the Trustor's bank. Though the Trustor must pay regular interest to maintain formalities, whether or not he actually pays off the *principal* is legally immaterial.

He can even borrow on top of borrowing, that is, borrowing to pay past interest. Brazil does exactly this with the IMF and Chase Manhattan *et al* every year. Although Brazil's debt is still kept on the books as current (since the formalities of interest payments are being observed), everybody knows the principal will *never* be repaid. We, too, can play this game.

The necessity of foreign entities
You must learn to think internationally. It will be the only way to survive financially in the next century.

Domestic entities
own little or nothing, but generate high expenses to their foreign counterparts, thus resulting in little or no taxable income. They operate as hollow "front men" in the hostile environment of taxation, regulation, lawsuits, etc.--offering little to tax, attach, or seize (no assets).

Foreign entities
own nearly everything. They lease and lend *to* their domestic counterparts at high rates which creates high U.S.A. expenses and thus low accounting profit. (Remember, the revenue of one firm is an expense for the other.) Properly structured, these foreign entities can reap most of an operation's overall profit, in tax-free form.

The overall structure
Let's say that I wanted to restructure a personally-held factory into a network of foreign and domestic trusts. The main goal is that no entity deriving taxable income should own property. That way, if the IRS has a bone with one of your income entities, it's got no assets to seize--everything is *leased*. Here's a rough example; international entities are underlined.

Example International
owns your personal domicile, furnishings, paintings, antiques, jewelry, clothing, etc. EI has utterly no business presence or activity within the U.S. and is in no way connected with any business operation of the empire. EI merely owns your personal tangibles and doesn't risk your personal wealth by entangling it with business ventures (which are subject to taxes and lawsuits). Unless EI actually sells some asset for a capital gain, it derives no income and pays no state/federal income tax.

Example Investments International
owns all patents, copyrights and business investments (stock, bonds, gold, silver, collectibles, etc.). EII has no business presence or activity within the U.S. Regarding U.S. income,

EII makes only *passive* income (i.e., nonactive: interest, capital gain royalties). **Foreign passive income from U.S. sources can be *nontaxable.***

EII is also your investment banker. It receives all empire venture capital and subsequently lends out (with surcharge) the necessary capital to the other **Example** entities. This creates a greater tax write-off interest expense for domestic **Example** firms, and **EII**'s interest revenue (which naturally includes a profit for brokering these loans) is passive income.

Since maintaining large cash balances in U.S. banks is extremely risky (bank failures, IRS assessments, etc.) and offers no financial privacy in exchange for anemic service, the bulk of your business cash should be kept *outside* the rapacious grasp of the Federal Government--meaning in offshore banks. The U.S. accounts of domestic entities should maintain balances just sufficient to cover routine disbursement, *and no more.* As soon as excess funds arrive, they are expatriated offshore in the form of business expenses (interest, leasing and consulting fees, etc.). If a cash crunch occurs, **EII** will naturally be only too happy to lend the needed funds--at a stiff rate, of course.

Example Properties International

owns all business land and buildings (foreign and domestic), and leases all domestic properties *in toto* (in totality) to **Example Properties U.S.A.** under one lease. To my understanding, a mere single lease does not constitute *"effective trade or commerce"* within the U.S. and would be nontaxable.

Example Properties U.S.A.

leases your domestic properties *from* **EPI** and subleases them to your domestic firms. **EPU** would make income.

Example Leasing International

owns all shop/office equipment, business vehicles, etc. and leases such *in toto* to its domestic counterpart **ELU**. (Notice the identical relationship between **EPI/EPU** and **ELI/ELU**.)

Example Leasing U.S.A.

leases all above equipment *from* **ELI** and subleases it to your domestic firms, independent contractors, etc.

Example Manufacturing U.S.A.

leases property from **EPU** and equipment from **ELU**. It then buys raw materials, contracts out any necessary operations, manufactures its products and wholesales to your domestic and international distributors.

Example Sales U.S.A.

neither owns property/equipment, nor manufactures products, but merely purchases product from **EMU** and serves as origin of all sales inside the U.S.A. **ESU** markets and sells in America, and contracts out certain sales, administrative and clerical responsibilities.

Example Sales International

operates as the origin for all sales *outside* the U.S.A. **ESI** has no business presence or activity within the U.S.A., but may have a conduit "information office" (and officers) to liaise with domestic firms. **ESI**'s revenue must come solely from *foreign* sources, or else it could be subject to U.S. income tax.

ESI purchases its product from **ESU** at just over cost, thus reducing the domestic (taxable) profit of **ESU**.

Overview of the empire

To summarize, there are nine firms: four domestic and five foreign. It is no mere coincidence that none of the four domestic firms (**EPU, ELU, EMU, ESU**) own any assets beyond the "shirt on their backs" (if that!). Remember, these domestic firms serve as frontline troops in a hostile legal and regulatory environment. If they are successfully breached by government or lawyers, *there exists no spoils for the "victor."* As empty, replaceable vessels, they could savaged by the IRS or a court judgment *with no appreciable detriment to the empire's overall net worth or operations.* Clone the destroyed company and get back up on line in a day!

The five foreign firms own everything, without being *"effectively connected with the conduct of a trade or business within the United States"*--therefore tax-proof and lawsuit-proof. Merely owning domestic property or maintaining an "information office" does *not* constitute business activity, according to the IRS.

Growth is *encouraged,* not hampered

Such a structure will not hamstring your journey and works *with* you, not against you. Once set up, you'll never have to revamp the thing as you grow. Just add on the necessary modules.

Under this arrangement, responsibilities are clearly defined and separated. Moreover, instead of these duties being under one corporate roof, they operate under their own respective autonomy.   This allows every uniquely talented individual to work with little interference.

By the modular separation of ownership and control, capital and risk, expense and revenue, profit and taxes, these items may be strategically placed.   This in turn offers unparalleled flexibility, efficiency, versatility, impregnability and maneuverability. Operating similarly to the human body, this empire is organically synergistic.   The normal cycles of internal growth and atrophy are smoothly handled occasions.

Its many advantages:
- ☞ Unmatched tax benefits
- ☞ Defensible contractor status (avoiding "employer" status)
- ☞ Compartmentalization of liability
- ☞ Separation of assets from lawsuit-vulnerable firms
- ☞ Superior vehicle for financial growth and retention
- ☞ Unbeatable privacy from outsiders (gov't., competitors, etc.)
- ☞ Minimized overlapping of personnel
- ☞ Reduced risk/effect of embezzlement and industrial espionage
- ☞ Smooth incorporation of new investors and partners
- ☞ Streamlined administrative automation
- ☞ Bottlenecks within/between modules quickly identified/opened
- ☞ Allows parallel modules (factory and sales) of intercompetition
- ☞ Organic/Synergistic

What are the risks?
As this structure is quite judgment-proof, the more likely threat I see to all this is from the IRS.   Even though tax-avoidance through trusts *is* legal, the IRS doesn't like it.   The IRS might have these areas of contention:

Utter absence of employees and total use of contractors.
Successfully classifying your independent contractors as employees for tax purposes would clearly mean the most money (and future control) for the IRS.   I don't see an IRS victory on this because: independent DBA (doing business as) craftsmen would be renting tools/equipment from **ELU** by the day, working unsupervised to the order specifications of **ESU**, while selling their finished components to **EMU** by lot.   Therefore, they meet the IRS criteria for independent contractors:

They have a regular place of business *outside* your office, with phone, bank accounts, multiple customers, etc.

They work on their *own* time.

They bill by the *job,* not by the hour/week/month. If they don't meet the contracted quality/quantity, they aren't paid.

They don't use *your* tools or equipment, as **ESU** and **EMU** own none and **ELU** is not involved in manufacture or sales.

They do *not* work under the direct supervision of **EMU**.

Intentionally meager profitability of U.S.A. firms through offshore cost structuring.

The huge multinational corporation are experts at the pricing game. Just learn their techniques. There is probably a *de facto* minimum markup which the domestic firm needs to charge to avoid alerting the IRS.

Mere existence and use of the offshore trusts themselves.

Properly formed and maintained, foreign trusts are nearly unassailable. Strict formalities must be observed, of course, but trusts are amazing flexible devices. Thousands of firms are operating along similar lines to my example; these are *not* uncharted waters.

It is important to create the structure *first,* so that the new companies are the *original* contractors and equipment purchasers. If the foreign trust network is created *after* the company has substantial assets and revenue, the IRS has been known to apply a punitive 35% excise tax on the value of assets *transferred* into foreign entities, or even disallow the new structure. Avoid any subsequent transfer of assets and income by having the empire in operation from Day 1. If the empire has *always* owned the assets from the beginning, then no transfer ever took place, therefore no transfer tax can apply.

In summary

I realize that forming and running many entities seems complex and perhaps daunting, but this example was for a factory. Most people, however, are likely to need only three trusts. Admittedly, the initial cost of this empire will be higher and will demand more time and paperwork to maintain. However, once set up, it will practically run itself. And, your extra effort and expense will be munificently rewarded by an infrastructure proven remarkably effective in supporting growth and defending your net worth.

If you continue under a sole-proprietorship or partnership form of operation, not only will you *not* be able to grow painlessly, but you will remain defenseless to those ever circling

---

buzzards of envy--government, lawyers and the masses. Right now, a single malicious lawsuit or punitive tax assessment could wipe you out.

With your children's' future at stake, the family's net worth must be protected in these perilous times of rampaging envy. By erecting a network of protective trusts, you not only safeguard your own retirement, but the rightful inheritance to your children. They will immeasurably benefit, not only by their inheritance, but by the *education* in the crucial knowledge of capital protection through common-law trusts. This priceless knowledge will be worth more to them than even their inheritance itself. Without this knowledge (and its practiced application) the next generation can neither hope to *achieve* any personal fortune, nor expect to *retain* it.

Only the courageously wise will prosper during the coming years. The timid I.Q. 100's will, at best, merely exist day by day in Neanderthal boredom with the approximate dignity and freedom of yoked oxen.

Become your *own* expert

There are many charlatans out there, so you'll have to gain your *own* knowledge to protect yourself. The primary question you should always ask yourself is, *"Can I trust the Trustee?"* A larcenous trustee will make worthless any trust's fine paperwork and clean out your assets. *Cuidado.*

Order a copy of *Knowledge=Freedom* (see Chapter 20) and check out the asset protection listings. Avoid anybody skittish about fully showing and explaining their paperwork. If they won't show you a sample indenture, it's probably because they copied somebody else's and retypeset it as their own. **Finally, *never* sign what you don't *clearly* understand.** Good luck.

FINAL THOUGHTS

I hope that *Bulletproof Privacy* has given you at least a good head start on low-key living. Privacy is not some theoretical legal approach. Privacy is real-world. It works.

Going over your privacy measures

While *anybody* can be found out with sufficient time, money and effort, with this information you probably will not be *worth* so much time, money and effort. Especially since you:

have a street-addressed mail drop as your "official" address.

Backed up by the R.R. box # ploy, the mail drop is what you give all government agencies: voter's registration, driver's license and vehicle registration, social security, IRS and state tax authorities, schools, VA, passport application, professional licenses, hunting/fishing licenses, and courts. All private firms get it too: insurance companies, employment agencies, doctors, credit bureaus, banks and financial institutions, car dealers, mail-order firms, clubs and organizations, and churches.

You *never* give out your *real* address except to good friends. You never receive mail there, except utility bills.

have a secret P.O. box for private correspondence.

That way, since your friends never write to your official address, they can't be discovered through a mail cover.

have a voice mail number as your "home phone."

This is given to all acquaintances, agencies and companies which allegedly have a "need to know"--such as: banks, car rental companies, airlines, video rental stores, classified ads, etc. As you don't even *have* a home phone (or if you do, it's not in your name), a major source of privacy loss is avoided. You check your voice mail from irregular pay phones at varied times.

have a cell phone with VM and pager notification for friends.

You receive and make only local calls to select friends whom you deeply trust. Ideally, your phone is always turned off and your friends page you with a code saying, *"It's 'me'--turn on your phone in XX minutes and I'll call you."* That way, your cellular bill only shows numberless incoming calls. Your conversations are very discreet, knowing full well that the cellular provider digitally records them in case of billing disputes.

You *never* make cell calls to government agencies, mailorder firms or local businesses. You *never* call the plumber, as that would be a trigger to where you live. You *never* make longdistance calls from this number, not even toll-free calls (which create a billing record and ANI information by the callee).

use prepaid calling cards from pay phones for long-distance calls.

Each area (private, business, alias, etc.) of your life has its own card and block of pay phones. (*Ideally*, you never use the same pay phone more than once.) You store the numbers in a PDA or notebook computer, burn the cards, and "wipe" (better than mere "delete") the numbers when used up.

have no checking account and credit cards, or use them carefully.

You *never* pay for sensitive or house-related items by check or credit card. Travel, gun-related, regular locale items are paid always with cash. Payments sent by mail are with M.O.'s. Let your checking and credit card accounts reveal nothing but purposeful misinfo about your life.

are not a borrower-slave, but a sovereign.

You *can* live without credit. Consumer credit is a postWWII phenomenon which has largely sapped this country of its diligence, financial good stewardship and ability to delay gratification. A nation of savers has become one of borrowers with negative net worth. Dwell on how much the government and big corporations know about you through your own, voluntarily filled out credit applications. Be hidden and free--pay with cash. If you can't buy it outright, then you don't deserve it.

hide your wealth in gold/silver, guns, food and usable assets.

Knowing what a house of cards the modern financial world is, you resist the lure of interest-bearing mutual funds, CD's, etc. Such is based on interconnected *debt*, not productivity. Storing wealth in useful commodities instead of phantom paper credits assures your private material independence.

place your visible, vulnerable assets in trusts.

You own nothing, yet control everything. You are judgment resistant, private, and your heirs avoid probate.

With an overall privacy posture such as *this,* you would not likely be worth the time, money, and effort to find. Every commonly helpful avenue is in actuality a *cul-de-sac.* Addresses, phone numbers, vehicle registration, credit cards--they all lead *nowhere.* Tee, hee.

Some final advice

Before closing, I want to reiterate the vital points.

Establish your own cash-oriented business.

This not only directly enhances your privacy, but you will avoid the forthcoming "citizen workers' national I.D. card" to be demanded of all *"employees."* Entrepreneurs will (for a while) escape such a Nazi/Soviet measure.

As more and more people use DigiCash (the only *truly* anonymous, double-blind form of digital payment for Internet purchases), a separate, private, parallel economy will emerge. All freedom-loving individuals simply must be a part of it.

Stock a self-sufficient RV and park it in the country.

Americans have emasculated themselves because of their wealth--they don't want to "make waves" for fear of losing their stuff. A partial solution: geographically diversify your things. Don't have everything on the line at one public address. As author Dresden James put it, *"Better a sovereign in squalor than a slave in splendor!"* Amen. Material wealth is a *means,* not an end. Don't let the tail wag the dog.

Don't sell your excess items at garage sales for pennies. Put the old TV, kitchen stuff, clothes, etc. in your country RV.

Create your escape line far in advance.

Think of it as insurance. If you must someday ditch everything, you should have already blazed the trail ahead of you. You'll need cash, gold/silver coins, guns, camping gear, second ID (with a 2nd passport, if possible), clothes, vehicles, safe houses and friends, disguise equipment, prearranged meeting points and fall-back plans, and practice drills for the family.

While you might get away with a bit of laziness or carelessness with the *first* layer of privacy--take utterly no chances with the escape line and second layer. Be especially sure not to create any "triggers" with your phone and credit card records. Keep your mouth shut--don't brag or hint around.

I personally live on less than a third of my assets. The rest are hidden and sprinkled about. That way, I'm more free to bolt since I know I'll always have another place of mine to go. I won't feel pressured to make a foolish stand at my "castle". I'd rather have many houses than one "castle".

If they ever come for you, *your house and things are gone already.* **You *won't* be able to hold back the focused resources of the U.S. Government.** (Ask the Weavers or the Branch Davidians.) Put up a good fight to buy yourself time, and escape to fight another day. Randy Weaver had *eighteen months* to create an escape plan for himself and his family. Once the first ambush was over, the Weavers still had several hours to split while the courageous U.S. Marshals were either running away or huddling in the woods.

Adopt a more basic and private life in the country.

Actually, wealth is more properly measured by that which we can do *without*--not by the things we have. Wealth is in *being* and *knowing*--not in having.

Move to the country if you can. The people are better, the environment is healthier and you'll rediscover your family. A voice mail number and postal drop will accomplish the same for you in the country as it does in NYC.

Drop your excess "friends" and acquaintances.

Write down a list of your "friends" and decide who would risk their lives and property for you. Who would stand by you in some smear campaign or punitive legal action? Who would hide you in their home if you ever became a fugitive from injustice? Who can be trusted to keep their mouth shut? Who is solid and dependable, not flighty or nervous?

Check off your *quality* people and drop the rest. You must immediately lower your social vulnerability.

Get your guns, gold and groceries--*now!*

These staples have no substitute. Without them, you must become utterly dependent on and submissive to the Corporate International Socialists for your existence.

Merely owning guns is *not enough*. You must also have the *training* and the *courage* to defend yourself.

Unless you've been to a *quality* defensive shooting school, you really have no idea what you *don't* know about using a gun to protect yourself. There is simply no substitute for having the best training doctrine ingrained in your muscle memory. During a lethal confrontation, you will not be able to *reliably* present your weapon and neutralize the threat--unless you have been *trained* to do so. **If you have not trained, you've in effect trained yourself to do *nothing*.** And *nothing* is exactly what you'll do, even if you've got the best gear and weapons.

While there are many schools, most of them pretty good, I know of no better training and facilities than Clint Smith's **Thunder Ranch** in Texas (830-640-3138). The courses are five days long and tuition is Ø900. Including travel, lodging, ammo, etc. each course is a Ø2,000 experience. I *strongly* recommend taking *at least* Handgun 1 and Urban Rifle 1. Why a *rifle* class? Because a pistol is merely a weapon you use to fight your way *back* to your *rifle* (which you *shouldn't* have left behind). After these first two classes, take Handgun 2 & 3, and Urban Rifle 2.

Yeah, it's a *lot* of money, but what use is that money *saved* if some dirtbag blows you away because you wouldn't pay for quality training? Don't fool yourself into believing that shooting stationary targets from a bench at the gun range is "training." How *often* are people assaulted, while sitting behind a table, by non-moving paper targets 25 yards away? You see my point.

Get *serious*. Sell some superfluous guns; you can only shoot one at a time, and you need the training more. Get down to Thunder Ranch while it's still *legal* to go. **Such training will be soon deemed *"terrorist"* or *"paramilitary."*** This may be your last year to go. Cops and feds go to Thunder. You can and should, too. In no time in history have civilians had the freedom to own and carry firearms as we do, with such excellent training available. Neither will last forever.

Support freedom-fighting organizations--*today!*

Larry Pratt's *"No Compromise"* Gun Owners of America springs to mind. Join the GOA (www.gunowners.org) and get on their email alert. (Use a discreet phone number.) To learn of many other liberty lovers, order a copy of *Knowledge = Freedom* (see the next chapter). We may not be able to turn this mess around, but we can certainly slow it down and increase our size.

The OKBomb(s) trials will be *pivotal* for Liberty.
These are scheduled for mid-1997. This book will have already been out for months. Whatever the verdicts, one thing is certain: either the Patriots or the Federal Government will be the loser, and things will quickly roll downhill thereafter. Several points seem already established:

The feds not only *knew* of the bombing plan, but had persons on the inside (as they did in the Trade Center bombing).

The feds also could have *prevented* the bombing, but delayed arrests for greater drama and publicity.

The evidence points more towards contact high-explosive than airburst, low pressure ammonium-nitrate fuel oil (ANFO). The alleged ANFO device was, according to virtually every bomb expert interviewed, *too far away* and 3-5 times *too slow* to shatter those reinforced concrete columns. Also, there was utterly no ANFO residue left--either on the ground in unignited ammonium nitrate prills, or on the building as ANFO soot, or in the air as ammonia fumes. Ted Gunderson, retired FBI Special Agent in Charge of the L.A. office, said that an ANFO device in a parked truck couldn't have done the damage. This was also confirmed by Brig. General Partin (USAF, Retired), an expert on weapons and SDI.

Irrefutable seismographic evidence from University of Oklahoma recordings prove that *two* "events" (explosions) occurred at 9:04AM. Many earwitnesses recall two blasts.

Parents and relatives of victims who publicly demanded to know *"Where was the ATF?"* were told to *"shut up!"* Most ATF agents escaped unscathed--they weren't in the building.

Rescue efforts on 19 April were halted, while injured were trapped and dying, to locate and remove secret ATF files.

The feds were in an awful hurry to demolish the building *less than a month* after 19 April, despite the opposition of Congress. The carted-off wreckage is still under guard. (What are they so nervous about? What are they hiding?)

Timothy McVeigh, while likely having considerable complicity in the bombing, seems to have been carefully set up to take the full rap. After blowing up a building and killing 169 people, would *you* get into a getaway car with no license plate, not to mention allow yourself to be disarmed and arrested by a single highway patrolman?

And what about John Doe #2 with the foreign accent? After the most intensive manhunt in American history, the feds say *"Oh, never mind about him. He's nothing to do with it."* John Doe #2 has been identified by some as the enigmatic, young German Army Captain Andreas Strassmeir. Strassmeir has admitted to working as a BATF infiltrator of Elohim City, described as a Christian Identity compound near Muldrow, Oklahoma. Another Elohim City plant, Michael Brescia, worked with Strassmeir and even shared a house with him. Strassmeir is back in his native Berlin, and Brescia can't be found.

In short, the bombing seems to have been an FBI/BATF counterintelligence operation gone bad. McVeigh and Nichols were probably at least *in part* set up for it. I pray that this comes out in the trials to blacken the face of the Government. Whether or not Americans will truly *care* remains to be seen.

Throw an utter *fit* over any biometric national I.D. plan.

This scheme is *the* prerequisite to the final tyranny. We must defeat this "on the beaches" and not allow a bridgehead for the following invasion. Don't be polite or reasonable with Congress--be ugly, unreasonable and vicious! It will be our last chance to fight *politically.* If we lose, politics will be irrelevant.

We cannot allow a centralized, biometric I.D. system to exist. It will strangle our last liberties to death. Any such equipment should be destroyed--from readers in squad cars to microwave nodes to central databanks.

ONE WARM AND FUZZY WORLD

Men have labored together to join the world under centralized control since the Tower of Babel. Scattered people, language, and knowledge have been progressively uniting for thousands of years. Organizers of this now proclaim humanity to have arrived at the dawn of a "New Age."

> *This agenda is nothing less than the complete revolutionizing of the very foundations of not only America but the entire world. Such a plan calls for the total restructuring of planetary civilization into an enlightened One World Federation in which national boundaries and sovereignty are secondary, and "planetary citizenship" in the "global village" is the order of the day. This* [conspiracy] *offers a world in desperate need a grand solution to profound global problems. Apparent world peace and unprecedented opportunities...are to be unveiled. Herein lies the Antichrist's last temptation, offered to all the world.*
> -- Randall Baer; *Inside the New Age Nightmare*

People, language, and knowledge are no longer, through a neural silicon net, scattered. The last, real obstacle is the lingering nation-state--America, in particular.

> _It is evident that the danger of a communist domination over the world has been replaced by a globalist and mercantile domination. This ideology aims at world government by a small financial oligarchy, backed by the United Nations and the various international enforcement agencies. The proponents of this new world domination consider the nations of the world as their principal enemies._ (In my _Hologram of Liberty_, I discuss how Hamiltonian Federalists saw the state sovereignties as enemies of the new Constitutional Nation. **The states were cunningly eroded into nothing just like the nations are today being eroded by the U.N.** BTP) _It is their aim to weaken them and then destroy the nations. Once this is accomplished, then will come the reign of "Big Brother"..._
>
> **_Let us not be mistaken about this: We are witnessing a veritable conspiracy to create a global power that would deprive the people of their national independence._** _I believe that the nation is still the best political framework to ensure the defense, the independence, the security, the identity, the freedom and the prosperity of people._
>
> -- Jean-Marie Le Pen, head of France's _National Front Party_

"We're so sane...we're insane."

A very good friend made this comment during a discussion of our national predicament. This is one of the most cogent descriptions of the Freedom Movement I've ever heard.

To elaborate, insanity is a functional disassociation with reality. Conversely, sanity means a firm, clear grasp on how things truly are. However, what's really going on is so sneaky and covert, it bears little semblance to what I term the "public reality." To the public, we Patriots have little hold on ("public") reality and we are "delusional, paranoid and militant." We're _so_ sane that we're _insane_. A liberal democrat reading my books would conclude that I'm quite nuts.

As William Allen White put it, _"There is no insanity so devastating in man's life as utter sanity."_ Utter sanity recognizes the utter _insanity_ of this world. Our political systems are driven by fear, ignorance, and power lust. But...

> _We go by the major vote, and if the majority is insane, the sane must go to the hospital._
> -- Horace Mann

Clear thinking and hardy personal responsibility will always be outnumbered by the brute beasts of humanity. America had a miraculous window of opportunity for its birth. Those conditions which led to its independence and growth no longer exist.

> *One of the best ways to get yourself a reputation as a dangerous citizen these days is to go about repeating the very phrases which our founding fathers used in the great struggle for independence.*
> -- Charles A. Beard

Thus, the necessity for this book. If the national soil is no longer fertile ground for liberty, dignity and honest success, then we must quietly and quickly create our own "gardens."

> **And the rulers knew not whither I went, or what I did...**
> -- Nehemiah 2:16

Introducing...Patriot Light!
A third less courage than the regular Patriot!

I speak of a respected newsletter writer who has become overly skittish. When his newsletter recently came under the beady scrutiny of some liberal rag and he was falsely linked to "hate" groups (whatever *those* are), he freaked. Although he has for years denounced the evil deeds of our government and advocated physical preparedness, he's now spooked.

He is frantically disassociating himself from the untax, sovereignty, and militia movements (which he's never championed) with a new disclaimer in his newsletters. According to an employee, he *"is like a kid who calls the schoolyard bully names from a distance and then retracts it all when confronted."*

Can he truly believe that this back-peddling will influence the feds--*"Oh, gee, sorry! We were all wrong about you!"* **The feds will not tolerate "Patriot *Lights*"--and neither will the Patriots.** They will be welcome nowhere, spewed out for being lukewarm (Rev. 3:15-6).

I say these things in the hope of shocking him out of his panic. This man, whom I consider a friend, is crumpling at the first *"Boo!"* Why? Because he doesn't want to lose his property. **We are born without assets and we die without assets.** There are no luggage racks on hearses. What matters is *how you lived your life!* Assets are merely the *tools* used to live an honorable life. When honor is forsaken for assets, honor is lost forever. **Assets are *expendable*. Character isn't.**

There were no "Patriot *Lights*" on 4 July 1776

The price paid by many signers of the Declaration of Independence was truly staggering:

Francis Lewis had his home burned and his wife tortured by the British for two years. She died shortly after her release.

John Hart's home was looted and burned, his ailing wife died and his 13 children were scattered. He eluded capture by sleeping in caves.

The 1,000 acre estate of **Lewis Morris** was ransacked and burned. His home was destroyed, his cattle butchered, and his family driven off.

Richard Stockton was captured, imprisoned, and repeated beaten at the brink of starvation. His home was destroyed, his papers burned.

Carter Braxton saw virtually every merchant ship he owned sunk or captured. He was forced to sell off his land.

Thomas McKean *"was hunted like a fox"* and was once *"compelled to move my family five times in a few months."*

Thomas Nelson, Jr. led 3,000 Virginia militia against the British. Redcoats took refuge in his own home, so he turned a cannon on it.

DON'T GET SKITTISH!

Posterity! You will never know how much it cost [us] *to preserve your freedom. **I hope you will make good use of it.***
    -- John Quincy Adams

If we are left alone, either by truce or by inefficiency, so be it. However, *if,* despite our best efforts for peaceful privacy, we be hounded unmercifully, if we be dragged away for the ID chip implants--**then give 'em fang and claw.**

I will not compromise, I will not grovel, I will not toady at the feet of mammon. I will not forsake my conscience and standards to the "value relative" sea of humanity. I will give every man his due. I will honor my word to my own hurt--and if these be insufficient grounds to be left alone, then somebody will have a seething problem on their hands.

I *will* be left alone to cause no harm. I hereby pledge to you my life, my fortune, and my sacred honor that I will die on my feet before I ever live on my knees. What about *you?*

Every man dies. Not every man really lives.
    -- William Wallace; *Braveheart*

ALTERNATIVE
SOURCES

To learn more on freedom-related matters, there are thousands of books available from several mail-order companies. Most of these below demonstrate excellent judgment by carrying my *You & The Police!* (and probably *Bulletproof Privacy*, too). I'd get all their catalogs and plan on dropping at least Ø1,000 in orders. Our time down here is vaporously short, and we simply won't live the years necessary to learn this uncommon sense firsthand. Many of these books are comparatively expensive (usually 10¢ or more per page), but keep in mind that this is *eccentric* stuff. For example, do you really expect to find Erwin S. Strauss's *How To Start Your Own Country* at Waldenbooks? Support these mail-order companies while we *can*--before they're put out of business by statute, tax audits, etc.

Here they are, in no particular order. Prices for catalogs range from free to Ø5. Underlined names carry my books.

MAIL-ORDER BOOK CATALOGS

Laissez-Faire Books   800-326-0996

A Libertarian/Objectivist oriented, highly intellectual catalog company, they are to be highly commended for taking a chance on my screamingly street-savvy *You & The Police!* (Thanks Andrea!) While they don't have *too* many practical books, lovers of liberty need quality "food for thought."

Second Renaissance Books   800-729-6149

More Objectivist/Randian focused than Laissez-Faire.

Liberty Tree   800-927-8733
The book catalog by the Libertarian think-tank *The Independent Institute*. A good selection of erudite material. Thanks to David and Mary Theroux for featuring *You & The Police!*

Loompanics Unlimited   360-385-7471
With over 700 titles carried in its 190+ page catalog, if it's unusual, they'll have it. *Really* eccentric stuff. They've got books on *subjects* you didn't know existed.

Eden Press   800-338-8484
A smaller, but more personal, alternative book catalog company operated by Barry Reid (author of the *Paper Trip* books). Barry lives the life and walks the walk. A good source for privacy and ID material. The operation is family owned and operated, with the sweetest telephone staff you've ever heard.

Paladin Press   800-392-2400
They carry a bit on everything, especially weapons and tactics. Their video collection on martial arts training is quite good. (I recommend the Jim Grover shooting series.)

They were recently the target of an insipid, vicious lawsuit because a hired hit man used one of their books to commit murder. A federal judge (grudgingly) granted summary dismissal, which was appealed. Tragically, Paladin's insurance company settled just days before the appeal went to trial, and threw seven figures at the family.

Knowledge = Freedom   702-329-5968
This is the Freedom Movement's "Yellow Pages." With over 2,000 listings (alphabetized and cross-referenced by subject matter and state/city), this continually updated compendium is a labor of love by Dennis Grover. A must.

CPA Book Publishers   503-668-4941
They carry nearly *every* Patriot/Freedom book.

Information Exchange   800-346-6205
Good selection on a variety of topics.

The Resource Center   800-922-1771
Mostly books on financial privacy, trusts, foreign banking, passports, etc.

Bohica Concepts   360-497-7075
Good selection on freedom-oriented subjects.

Militia of Montana   406-847-2735
   Good selection of anti-NWO and survival books, gear, etc.

Cascadian Resource Center   503-343-5066
   Carries much forward-thinking material.

America West Catalog   406-585-0700
   Freedom books on varied subjects.

Bluestocking Press   800-959-8586
   Good source of home-schooling material.

NEWSLETTERS & MAGAZINES

The Anti-Shyster   **214-418-8993**
   Highly original legal contrarian magazine.

Full Disclosure   **800-633-3274**
   Fine material on privacy, anti-bugging, covert electronics.

The Free American   **505-423-3250**
   Timely and interesting.

American Survival Guide
   A quality magazine. Highly recommended.

Criminal Politics   **800-543-0486**
   The magazine of conspiracy politics.

Backwoods Home Magazine
   A must for you rural types.

Aid & Abet   **602-237-2533**
   Put out by *Police Against the New World Order* ministry.

Media Bypass Magazine
   Highly informative.

PRODUCTS

Phoenix Systems, Inc.   303-277-0305
   Interesting catalog of anti-bugging equipment, etc.

The Survival Center   800-321-2900
   Interesting survival gear.

U.S. Cavalry   800-777-7732
   Great color catalog.

Brigade Quartermasters   800-338-4327
   A competitor of the above.

Shomer-Tec   360-733-6214
   Interesting law enforcement and military equipment.

Major Surplus & Survival   800-441-8855
   Good selection of outdoor survival gear.

Cheaper Than Dirt   888-625-3848
   Excellent selection and prices. Great folks.
   Visit them online at www.cheaperthandirt.com

RECOMMENDED BOOKS

This Perfect Day, Ira Levin
   Sci-fi depiction of an eerie, smarmy dystopia where ID bracelets are the human control mechanism. Fascinating.

How To Achieve Personal and Financial Privacy
   Sweeping and highly detailed, however, this book by Mark Nestmann is more informative than instructive. ISBN 0-96279953-1-3. Possibly OP. Try 800-528-0559 or 702-885-2509.

Mark Skousen's Complete Guide to Financial Privacy
   I have the third revised edition of 1982. It's now quite dated in some areas, but has great classic information. I believe this was the last edition and is OP. ISBN 0-94322496-11-3.

anything by Thomas Perry
   Metzger's Dog, Butcher's Boy, The Big Fish, Dance For The Dead, Vanishing Act, and *Shadow Woman* all have a hunter/prey theme with lots of good privacy details and excellent psychological study. Highly recommended!

www.javelinpress.com

NOTE: Javelin Press is enjoying rapid growth, which may affect our address or pricing. Please verify both from our website *before* you send your order!

Prices each copy:	**Retail**	**<40%>**	**<44%>**	**<50%>**
Good-Bye April 15th! 8½"x11" 392 pp. 11/1992	1-2 copies **$40**	3-7 **$24**	8-15 **$22**	*case of 16 or more* **$20**
You & The Police! 5½"x8½" 168 pp. 2/2005	1-5 copies **$16**	6-37 **$10**	38-75 **$8.80**	*case of 76 or more* **$8**
Bulletproof Privacy 5½"x8½" 160 pp. 1/1997	1-5 copies **$16**	6-39 **$10**	40-79 **$8.80**	*case of 80 or more* **$8**
Hologram of Liberty 5½"x8½" 262 pp. 8/1997	1-5 copies **$20**	6-19 **$12**	20-39 **$11**	*case of 40 or more* **$10**
Boston on Surviving Y2K 5½"x8½" 352 pp. 11/1998	1-5 copies **$11**	6-17 **$10**	18-35 **$9**	*case of 36 or more* **$8**
Boston's Gun Bible 5½"x8½" 848 pp. 4/2002	1-2 copies **$28**	3-7 **$16.80**	8-15 **$15.70**	*case of 16 or more* **$14**
Molôn Labé! 5½"x8½" 454 pp. 1/2004	1-5 copies **$24**	6-13 **$14.40**	14-27 **$13.44**	*case of 28 or more* **$12**

Mix titles for *any* quantity discount. This is easiest done as ¼ case per title:
¼ case of: **GBA15!** 4   **Y&P!** 19   **BP** 20   **HoL** 10   **BoSY** 9   **BGB** 4   **ML!** 7

Shipping and Handling are *not* included!   Add below:

non-case S&H for *Good-Bye April 15th!*   *Boston's Gun Bible*   *Molôn* :
First Class (or UPS for larger orders) add: $6 for first copy, $2 each additional copy.

non-case S&H within USA for other titles (*i.e., Y&P!, BP, HoL,* and *BoSY*):
First Class (or UPS for larger orders) add: $5 for first copy, $1 each additional copy.

CASE orders (straight or mixed) UPS Ground: $25 west of the Miss.; $35 east.

Overpayment will be refunded in cash with order. Underpayment will delay order!
If you have questions on discounts or S&H, email us through our website.

These forms of payment *only:*

Cash (Preferred. Cash orders receive signed copies when available.)
payee blank M.O.s (Which makes them more easily negotiable.)
credit cards (Many of our distributors take them. See our website.)

Unless prior agreement has been made, *we do not accept and will return* checks, C.O.D.s, filled-in M.O.s, or any other form of tender. Prices and terms are subject to change without notice (check our website first). Please send paid orders to:

JAVELIN PRESS ● c/o P.O. Box 31B ● Ignacio, Colorado. (81137-0031)

Works by Boston T. Party:

Good-Bye April 15th!

The untaxation classic—crystal clear and sweeping. Copied, plagiarized, and borrowed from, but never equaled. The most effective and least hazardous untaxation guide. Proven over 12 years and thousands of readers!

392 pp. softcover (1992) $40 + $6 s&h (cash, please)

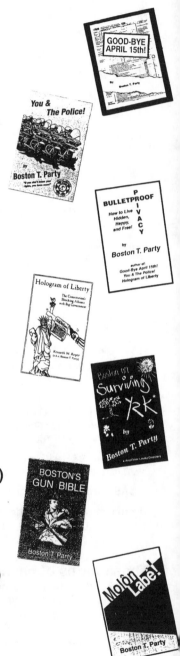

You & The Police! (revised for 2005)

The definitive guide to your rights and tactics during police confrontations. When can you *refuse* to answer questions or consent to searches? Don't lose your liberty through ignorance! This 2005 edition covers the *USA PATRIOT Act* and much more.

168 pp. softcover (2005) $16 + $5 s&h (cash, please)

Bulletproof Privacy

How to Live Hidden, Happy, and Free!

Explains precisely how to lay low and be left alone by the snoops, government agents and bureaucrats. Boston shares many of his own unique methods. The bestselling privacy book in America!

160 pp. softcover (1997) $16 + $5 s&h (cash, please)

Hologram of Liberty

The Constitution's Shocking Alliance
with Big Government   by Kenneth W. Royce

The Convention of 1787 was the most brilliant and subtle *coup d'état* in history. The nationalist framers *designed* a strong government, guaranteed through purposely ambiguous verbiage. Many readers say this is Boston's best book. A jaw-dropper.

262 pp. softcover (1997) $20 + $5 s&h (cash, please)

Boston on Surviving Y2K

And Other Lovely Disasters

Even though Y2K was Y2¿*Qué?* this title remains highly useful for all preparedness planning. **Now on sale for 50% off!** (It's the same book as The Military Book Club's *Surviving Doomsday*.)

352 pp. softcover (1998) only $11 + $5 s&h (in cash)

Boston's Gun Bible (new text for 2005)

A rousing how-to/*why*-to on modern gun ownership. Firearms are *"liberty's teeth"* and it's time we remembered it. Fully revised in 2002 with 10 new chapters. ***200+ new pages*** were added! Much more complete than the 2000 edition. No other general gun book is more thorough or useful! Indispensable!

848 pp. softcover (2002) $28 + $6 s&h (cash, please)

Molôn Labé!   (Boston's first novel)

If you liked *Unintended Consequences* by John Ross and Ayn Rand's *Atlas Shrugged*, then Boston's novel will be a favorite. It dramatically outlines an innovative recipe for Liberty which could actually work! A thinking book for people of action; an action book for people of thought. A freedom classic!

454 pp. softcover (2004) $24 + $6 s&h (cash, please)
limited edition hardcover $44 + $6 (while supplies last)

www.javelinpress.com
www.freestatewyoming.org

www.javelinpress.com

NOTE: Javelin Press is enjoying rapid growth, which may affect our address or pricing. Please verify both from our website *before* you send your order!

Prices each copy:	Retail	<40%>	<44%>	<50%>
Good-Bye April 15th! 8½"x11" 392 pp. 11/1992	1-2 copies **$40**	3-7 **$24**	8-15 **$22**	case of 16 or more **$20**
You & The Police! 5½"x8½" 168 pp. 2/2005	1-5 copies **$16**	6-37 **$10**	38-75 **$8.80**	case of 76 or more **$8**
Bulletproof Privacy 5½"x8½" 160 pp. 1/1997	1-5 copies **$16**	6-39 **$10**	40-79 **$8.80**	case of 80 or more **$8**
Hologram of Liberty 5½"x8½" 262 pp. 8/1997	1-5 copies **$20**	6-19 **$12**	20-39 **$11**	case of 40 or more **$10**
Boston on Surviving Y2K 5½"x8½" 352 pp. 11/1998	1-5 copies **$11**	6-17 **$10**	18-35 **$9**	case of 36 or more **$8**
Boston's Gun Bible 5½"x8½" 848 pp. 4/2002	1-2 copies **$28**	3-7 **$16.80**	8-15 **$15.70**	case of 16 or more **$14**
Molôn Labé! 5½"x8½" 454 pp. 1/2004	1-5 copies **$24**	6-13 **$14.40**	14-27 **$13.44**	case of 28 or more **$12**

Mix titles for *any* quantity discount. This is easiest done as ¼ case per title:
¼ case of: **GBA15!** 4   **Y&P!** 19   **BP** 20   **HoL** 10   **BoSY** 9   **BGB** 4   **ML!** 7

Shipping and Handling are *not* included!   Add below:

non-case S&H for *Good-Bye April 15th!*   *Boston's Gun Bible*   *Molôn* :
First Class (or UPS for larger orders) add: $6 for first copy, $2 each additional copy.

non-case S&H within USA for other titles (*i.e., Y&P!, BP, HoL,* and *BoSY*):
First Class (or UPS for larger orders) add: $5 for first copy, $1 each additional copy.

CASE orders (straight or mixed) UPS Ground: $25 west of the Miss.; $35 east.

Overpayment will be refunded in cash with order. Underpayment will delay order! If you have questions on discounts or S&H, email us through our website.

These forms of payment *only:*

Cash (Preferred. Cash orders receive signed copies when available.)
payee blank M.O.s (Which makes them more easily negotiable.)
credit cards (Many of our distributors take them. See our website.)

Unless prior agreement has been made, *we do not accept and will return* checks, C.O.D.s, filled-in M.O.s, or any other form of tender. Prices and terms are subject to change without notice (check our website first). Please send paid orders to:

JAVELIN PRESS ● c/o P.O. Box 31B ● Ignacio, Colorado. (81137-0031)

Works by Boston T. Party:

Good-Bye April 15th!

The untaxation classic—crystal clear and sweeping. Copied, plagiarized, and borrowed from, but never equaled. The most effective and least hazardous untaxation guide. Proven over 12 years and thousands of readers!

392 pp. softcover (1992) $40 + $6 s&h (cash, please)

You & The Police!   (revised for 2005)

The definitive guide to your rights and tactics during police confrontations. When can you *refuse* to answer questions or consent to searches?   Don't lose your liberty through ignorance! This 2005 edition covers the *USA PATRIOT Act* and much more.

168 pp. softcover (2005) $16 + $5 s&h (cash, please)

Bulletproof Privacy

How to Live Hidden, Happy, and Free!

Explains precisely how to lay low and be left alone by the snoops, government agents and bureaucrats. Boston shares many of his own unique methods. The bestselling privacy book in America!

160 pp. softcover (1997) $16 + $5 s&h (cash, please)

Hologram of Liberty

The Constitution's Shocking Alliance
with Big Government   by Kenneth W. Royce

The Convention of 1787 was the most brilliant and subtle *coup d'état* in history. The nationalist framers *designed* a strong government, guaranteed through purposely ambiguous verbiage. Many readers say this is Boston's best book. A jaw-dropper.

262 pp. softcover (1997) $20 + $5 s&h (cash, please)

Boston on Surviving Y2K

And Other Lovely Disasters

Even though Y2K was Y2¿Qué? this title remains highly useful for all preparedness planning. **Now on sale for 50% off!** (It's the same book as The Military Book Club 's *Surviving Doomsday*.)

352 pp. softcover (1998) only $11 + $5 s&h (in cash)

Boston's Gun Bible (new text for 2005)

A rousing how-to/*why*-to on modern gun ownership. Firearms are *"liberty's teeth"* and it's time we remembered it. Fully revised in 2002 with 10 new chapters. ***200+ new pages** were added!* Much more complete than the 2000 edition. No other general gun book is more thorough or useful! Indispensable!

848 pp. softcover (2002) $28 + $6 s&h (cash, please)

Molôn Labé!   (Boston's first novel)

If you liked *Unintended Consequences* by John Ross and Ayn Rand's *Atlas Shrugged*, then Boston's novel will be a favorite. It dramatically outlines an innovative recipe for Liberty which could actually work! A thinking book for people of action; an action book for people of thought. A freedom classic!

454 pp. softcover (2004) $24 + $6 s&h (cash, please)
limited edition hardcover $44 + $6 (while supplies last)

www.javelinpress.com
www.freestatewyoming.org